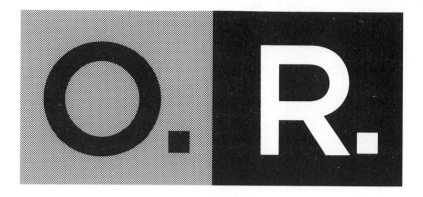

Also by B. D. Colen:

Karen Ann Quinlan
Born at Risk
Hard Choices
The Essential Guide to a Living Will
Mr. King, You're Having a Heart Attack (with Larry King)

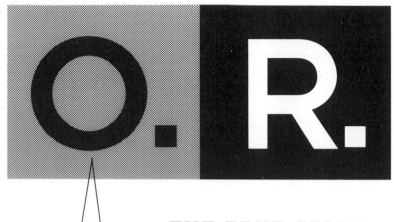

O. R.

THE TRUE STORY
OF 24 HOURS
IN A HOSPITAL
OPERATING ROOM

B. D. COLEN

A DUTTON BOOK

DUTTON
Published by the Penguin Group
Penguin Books USA Inc., 375 Hudson Street,
New York, New York 10014, U.S.A.
Penguin Books Ltd, 27 Wrights Lane,
London W8 5TZ, England
Penguin Books Australia Ltd, Ringwood,
Victoria, Australia
Penguin Books Canada Ltd, 10 Alcorn Avenue,
Toronto, Ontario, Canada M4V 3B2
Penguin Books (N.Z.) Ltd, 182–190 Wairau Road,
Auckland 10, New Zealand

Penguin Books Ltd, Registered Offices:
Harmondsworth, Middlesex, England

First published by Dutton, an imprint of New American Library, a division of Penguin
Books USA Inc.
Distributed in Canada by McClelland & Stewart Inc.

First Printing, April, 1993
10 9 8 7 6 5 4 3 2 1

 REGISTERED TRADEMARK—MARCA REGISTRADA

Library of Congress Cataloging-in-Publication Data
Colen, B. D.
    O.R. : the true story of 24 hours in a hospital operating room /
by B. D. Colen.
        p.   cm.
    ISBN 0-525-93518-5
    1. Surgery—Popular works. I. Title.
RD31.3.C64   1992
617'.9—dc20   92-26891
                                                        CIP

Printed in the United States of America
Set in New Baskerville
Designed by Leonard Telesca

For Nina Kohlmorgan and
the other special people at
Ocean Avenue Elementary School

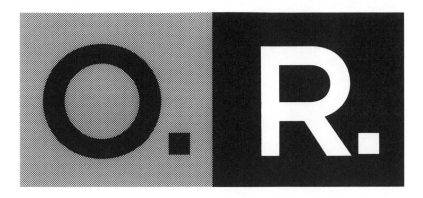

INTRODUCTION

Every year 10.9 million people are admitted to community hospitals in America for surgery. From the admitting department, where they promise to pay exorbitant charges their inadequate health insurance will never cover, they are taken to never-private rooms where they are tagged, gowned, and stripped of their dignity and individuality. From that moment on, they are patients and they are at the mercy of a system that seems designed for the comfort and convenience of everybody but them. They will be poked and prodded by all manner and variety of nurses, technicians, medical students, and residents. They may be rushed to high-tech laboratories for scheduled tests, only to be left for hours, shivering in chilled hallways, while some technician takes a lunch break. They may have blood drawn three times for the same series of tests, ordered by three different people. They may be awakened in the middle of the night to be given sleeping pills.

There have been hundreds of books written, from virtually all points of view, about this common experience known as hospitalization. Some of these books focus on the quality, or lack of quality, of the care received. Others focus on the obscene cost of that care. Some of these books

are funny. Some are sad. Many are frightening. Not a few
are angry. Most present varying views of the aspects of
hospitalization leading up to, or following, the one common experience shared by all 10.9 million surgical patients:

At some point in the hospital stay, all of those people
will be taken to a forbidden world called the O.R., where
a masked person they may have never seen before will put
them to sleep. They will awaken after the operation, with
no memory of it and no firsthand knowledge of anything
that was done to them while they lay in that windowless,
tile-walled room.

O.R. is the story of twenty-four hours in that world patients never see. But though this book reveals an unknown
world, it is not so much an exposé as a series of exposures,
an album of snapshots that together form a mosaic of life
in the operating room. *O.R.* is the story of what really
happens to patients when they have an operation. It is the
story of what surgeons, anesthesiologists, nurses, and the
various members of the operating room support staff do
when they go to work each day. On one level, it is a story
of routine, of attention to detail, of taking care of business
in much the same way that anyone who is a conscientious
worker takes care of business. On another level, however,
this is a story of secular miracles. For while we take modern
surgical achievements for granted, if we really stop to think
about what is accomplished on a daily basis in any operating
room, it is, indeed, miraculous.

For instance, we speak ever so casually of the more than
four hundred thousand coronary artery bypass operations
each year. Yet in each of those cases a person with a damaged heart is attached to a machine that does the work of
the heart and lungs, oxygenating and circulating the blood,
while surgeons saw open the patient's chest like a sidewalk
construction site, use drugs and near-freezing liquid to stop
the heart, cut it open, replace clogged arteries with arteries
removed from the patient's legs, restart the heart, and close

the chest. And the patient lives? It is neither naive nor exaggerated to call that miraculous.

We take it for granted that it is possible to surgically repair the face of a child who has a rough-edged hole where nose and mouth should be. Yet what that requires is that an artist who works in flesh wield knife and scissors, needle and thread, to turn one of nature's accidents into a normal child.

And it should boggle our minds that surgeons perform major abdominal surgery without cutting open the abdomen, operating instead by using fiber optics, a miniature videocamera and a TV monitor guiding their manipulation of miniaturized instruments inside the abdomen.

Those who perform these feats are not gods. Some of them are, in fact, surprisingly ordinary people, who lead ordinary lives outside the O.R. They are simply men and women with a great deal of education and training who possess egos so great that they are willing, even eager, to create gaping incisions in whole bodies in the belief that in wounding they can heal.

Welcome, then, to the world of the O.R. Once you have taken this journey, you will never again hear a reference to surgery without thinking about the twenty-four hours you spent here. There are two things about this trip that you may find somewhat disconcerting: the graphic descriptions of surgery and the general lack of physical descriptions of the men and women who people these sixteen operating rooms. The former are included not to shock, but because it is impossible to write about something not usually seen without describing it. The latter are generally omitted because the operating room is perhaps the only place in our society where the physical appearance of individuals is of absolutely no import.

I was governed by only three ground rules during the six weeks I spent in the sixteen rooms of the Main O.R. of

North Shore University Hospital, in Manhasset, New York.

The first, and most obvious, was that I not interfere in any way with patient care. The second was that I protect patient confidentiality. The third was that I honor any specific request, by patient or staff member, that the person not be included in this book. The surgeons who practice in the Main O.R., as well as the various staff members who work there, were told about my project and were given the option of cooperating with me or choosing not to, so long as they did not try to prevent others from participating. What these restrictions meant was that there were virtually no limitations placed on my ability to become one of the wall tiles in the Main O.R. I was given free access to all the operating rooms and was allowed to observe any procedure that interested me, ask any questions that occurred to me, and record any events and conversations that were within my sight and hearing. I was made welcome at the weekly M&M rounds, the Morbidity and Mortality meetings, at which the staff and attending surgeons discuss the week's most difficult cases, interesting cases, and those cases in which someone made a mistake. I was also invited to attend any departmental meetings that intrigued me.

The result of these rules and this access is a nonfiction book about a real place and the people who work there. Any time quotation marks are used, the words between those marks were spoken as I report them here, by the individual to whom I attribute them. The events in the book occurred as written, but they did not all occur in a single twenty-four-hour period, as I could not be in more than one room at any one time. That does not mean, however, that the twenty-four-hour period about which I have written is compiled from a collection of unusual, particularly dramatic cases. Instead, after reviewing dozens of daily surgery schedules, I constructed a typical day and night from the cases I had observed.

I have changed the names and altered minor personal details to protect the identity of all the patients about whom

I have written, even though some agreed to have their real names used. It was my feeling that, not understanding how completely they would be revealed during surgery, these patients could not give truly informed consent to being identified.

Similarly, I have changed the names of the nurses— other than head nurse Diana Potenza; the residents, except for Jim Sullivan, one of three chief residents; the technicians, other than Lee McFee; and the other support staff members in the O.R., with the exception of surgeon's assistant Dom DiCapua. It was my feeling that, while only one of these people asked that her name not be used, there might be the appearance of a certain element of coercion in the naming of those whose jobs and promotions depend upon hospital officials who approved this project.

That said, all the anesthesiologists and all but two of the surgeons named in the book are identified by their real names. Those exceptions are a plastic surgeon whom I named Jim Firstman, who came into the O.R. in the middle of a procedure and knew nothing of my project and had no opportunity to rationally consider his participation, and the pediatric surgeon whom I call Burt Parton, who came to the hospital to perform an appendectomy in the middle of the night and was similarly unable to consider the implications of my presence.

1

6:30 A.M. The hallways of the second-floor Main Operating Room area of North Shore University Hospital are still. Any moment now, the day nursing coordinator will take her place at the front desk, and a few minutes later the rush will begin, as the thirty members of the day-shift nursing staff arrive, preceding surgeons, anesthesiologists, technicians, and, when everyone else is ready, patients. On the south wall of the short hallway that forms part of the entrance area of the Main O.R., there is a small tan cork strip used for posting the nursing schedule. As one twenty-four-hour workday comes to an end and another is about to begin on this Thursday morning in late July, 1991, a handwritten note for the day shift hangs from the strip:

> Dear Staff,
> Very busy night. Instruments not picked for O.R.
> 6, 8, 9, 10. Basic instruments for other rooms. Emergency in progress in O.R. 6.
> Kathy.

In the argot of the Main O.R., an emergency is any pressing case that can't wait for the next opening in the regular operating schedule—anything from a patient who suffers a cardiac arrest in the middle of an angioplasty procedure in the cath lab, to something as mundane as an appendectomy or a compound fracture. But the mess in Room 6 is an emergency in any setting, a frantic-voice-on-a-telephone-calling-911 emergency, a skittering-along-the-technological-wall-separating-life-from-death emergency. The standard surgical consent form that has been taped to one of the room's pale green tile walls says it all. On the line reserved for the patient's signature, a resident has scrawled the words "Life or Death."

The mechanically ventilated body on the table in the center of the sixteen-by-twenty-foot room is that of a stocky, long-haired, forty-three-year-old white male with a tattoo of a snarling tiger on his left shoulder and a dagger on his right. The name SCOTT is tattooed on the patient's right hand, and there are two more tattoos on his thighs: on the right, a wonderfully executed grim reaper, complete with swinging scythe; and on the left, death throwing dice. The artwork has been the subject of some comment as the trauma team has struggled for the past seven hours to postpone Scott's meeting with the reaper. "You know Mike Garrett's two-tattoo rule, don't you?" the chief of anesthesia, Peter Walker, rhetorically asks the circulating nurse, who, as the person in charge of the functioning of the room, is attempting to catch up on the flood of paperwork being generated by the case under way.

"Two-tattoo rule?"

"Right. Mike says he won't ever give regional anesthesia to someone with two or more tattoos. They're lunatics and you can't depend on them to cooperate if they're awake during the procedure. Then there's the three-tattoo rule, of course," Walker adds, as he reaches up to adjust the flow from a bag of packed red blood cells hanging from a stand to the left of Scott's head. "If they have three tattoos you have to figure they're totally unreliable. You can't depend on anything they say."

The banter does not distract from the seriousness of the work in the blood-splattered room. Trauma surgeon Dan Reiner and Gil Martin, one of the three chief residents, seem aware of the joking, but continue their thus far vain attempt to fit a pile of intestines back into Scott's abdominal cavity. They had shoved his guts out of the way as they worked through the night to repair the damage done by the single thrust of a thin-bladed knife, held in the hand of "someone known to him." Scott's acquaintance knew what he was doing: his single thrust had pierced the duodenum, pancreas, inferior vena cava, and aorta.

"If this was a gunshot wound, the first thing the family would ask is, 'Did you get the bullet out?'" Reiner tells Martin.

"Yah, and if this was Jamaica Hospital, the first question would be, 'Did you get his sneakers? He was wearing new Pumps,'" the exhausted resident responds.

Walker has been working on his side of the "blood-brain barrier"—what anesthesiologists jokingly call the drape separating their work area from that of the surgeons—since being brought in on "second call" at 5:00 A.M., two hours before the scheduled start of his day. By that time the trauma team had already been at work on Scott for about five hours, and the anesthesiologist and the certified registered nurse anesthetist working the case needed a third pair of hands as they struggled to maintain something like fluid balance in their patient. It is now 7:06, and the chief of anesthesia is doing "housekeeping" chores, separating and counting the polystyrene bags that have held the 55 units of blood and fluid—the average adult body holds about 13—that Scott has already needed. He will receive a total of 57 before he leaves O.R. 6.

2

7:06 A.M. The morning rush is under way on Community Drive in Manhasset, New York, a few hundred feet west of the entrance to North Shore University Hospital. The heaviest traffic is in the two southbound lanes of this north-south artery, as commuters spill out of the gold coast suburbs surrounding the communities Jay Gatsby knew as East Egg and West Egg, onto the Long Island Expressway and into Manhattan, about seventeen miles to the west.

It is so foggy this morning that the hospital's dominant feature, the mirrored façade of the nine-story Payson-Whitney Tower, is barely distinguishable from the gray-brown mist enveloping it. The line of cars inching its way off Community Drive onto the hospital grounds seems not so much to drive into the garage and various parking lots as to melt into them. And many of the 3,778 nurses, secretaries, janitors, administrators, lab technicians, attorneys, clerks, anesthesiologists, and several hundred of the 1,785 staff and attending physicians hurrying across the hospital grounds, perhaps more anxious to escape the already oppressive summer heat than they are to get to work, vanish in the mist, seemingly transported to another world.

In fact, any hospital is another world, constantly proclaiming itself a part of its community, while all who work in it, are served by it, visit it, or just view it from afar know that it is in some ways as distant from its immediate surroundings as the Brazilian rain forest. And like the rain forest, the hospital is truly a place of daily struggles between life and death, of languages known only to those who venture within, of hierarchies and pecking orders rarely understood by outsiders and often abhorred by those who observe them; a place full of rumors often born of betrayal, and of secrets held beyond the grave. Every year, about 5,500 independent lives will begin here, and about 1,100 will end.

Within this sprawling medical complex, which in less than forty years has grown from a 169-bed community hospital to a 755-bed teaching arm of Cornell University Medical College, lies the Main O.R. Located in space partly carved out of the hospital's original brick building, and partly out of the Payson-Whitney Tower so visible from the surrounding community, the Main O.R. is a world within a world, as foreign to many who have spent their entire careers at North Shore as is the hospital itself to those who have never entered its doors. To paraphrase an old hymn, in here there is no east or west, in here no night or day.

If, in the corridors and world beyond the Main O.R., clothes make the man or woman, here they provide anonymity and a false perception of equality: men and women alike dress in the same green or blue paper scrub suits, cover their hair with one of three styles of paper hats, and choose one of three styles of mask. Physical appearances are subsumed by role. Chief of surgery, environmental technician (janitor), scrub nurse, anesthesiologist: each is a pair of eyes set in a two-inch band of skin framed by green or blue paper. Later, between cases, sitting in the hopelessly overcrowded little room that serves as lounge, lunchroom, and meeting room for the Main O.R., one may notice a particular set of eyes and think, "My God! Where did she get all that long red hair?" Or, "A mustache? He's been operating here for a month already and I didn't realize he had a mustache." For in the hallways, storage areas, and sixteen operating rooms that make up its sterile area, the Main O.R. resembles a sort of high-tech version of a fundamentalist Moslem marketplace.

The customs, mores, and procedures of this world are foreign even to the vast majority of the hospital's physicians and nurses. Once a patient has entered the Main O.R. for a scheduled procedure, she is in the hands of the surgeons, anesthesiologists, and 4 percent of the hospital's employees who work here on the day shift. Not until they have done their work does she return to the care of her attending physician. And while nurses may rotate through other assignments in the hospital, they do not pass through these doors unless they have come to stay: nursing in the Main O.R. requires a six-month orientation and a good two to three years on the job before a nurse is truly comfortable here. Thus, even to many of those who work on the patient units immediately adjacent to it, this isolated environment that serves more than ten thousand patients each year remains what even its head nurse calls "the unknown place."

3

7:35 A.M. The so-called "sterile envelope" of the Main O.R. is a fourteen-thousand-square-foot area on the hospital's second floor encompassing 16 operating rooms, the Recovery Room, special equipment storage areas, the anesthesia storage room, and various spaces used to sterilize instruments and package them for use. The area is roughly M-shaped, with the operating rooms and the storage areas arranged along three, 150-foot-long, eight-foot-wide corridors, with shorter connecting hallways. An alcove with a scrub sink is set into the sides of the hallways between each pair of operating rooms, with the alcoves, and anyone using the sinks, fully exposed to all passing traffic. At this moment two residents stand talking at the sink between Rooms 5 and 6, their backs to the passing parade.

". . . So I reached up three inches beyond where he tied and I got the specimen and pulled it out," the senior resident is telling his junior, in a voice loud enough to be heard over the running water as the two scrub their hands and arms to the elbows. "Sure it was bloody, so what? You tie it off and close. But Johnson was all upset. 'You got my uterine artery,' he says. 'Yah, I got your uterine,' I tell him, 'but it was three inches past your tie . . .'"

The two surgeons-in-training laugh raucously and walk away, their drying hands held up before them in the air. They make no note of, in fact they are totally unaware of, a woman lying on her back on a stretcher less than ten feet away in the hallway. She has an IV in her arm and a nasogastric tube running into her nose. But it is clear by the horrified expression on her face that she has heard every word the residents have said.

4

7:59 A.M. Scrub nurse Kathleen Kerr stands on the tips of her toes, stretching to reach the switches on the three round light fixtures above the operating table in Room 1A. The twenty-two lamps in the fixtures bathe the operating table in 1,100 watts of hot, white light, wiping all the color from Lillian Paskow's already pale skin. The fifty-three-year-old woman is lying naked on her back on the table, her elbows and heels cradled in blue foam rubber to prevent damage to the nerves that run through them, her legs encased in opaque "compression stockings," inflatable plastic wraps designed to prevent blood clots. Anesthesiologist Jonathan Singer has already intubated Paskow, and the endotracheal tube he slid past her larynx into her trachea is now attached to tubing connected to the mechanical ventilator breathing for her. Singer gave her Versed, a powerful chemical cousin of Valium that will ensure that Paskow remembers nothing from the time she was given the drug until Singer awakens her at the end of the procedure. Then he used the drug propofol to induce sleep, and he maintains sleep and blocks pain by giving Paskow nitrous oxide—laughing gas—and narcotics.

As the nurses cover Paskow's body with paper surgical

drapes, Dr. Michael Setzen places a blue drape from ear to ear, across her forehead, covering her eyes. Setzen uses a scissorlike surgical clamp to secure the drape and then begins palpating the patient's neck, feeling the outline of the hard malignant mass growing on her vocal cords. Using a disposable marking pen, he places five black dots on the skin above each of her carotid arteries, draws a small, faint V at the top of her sternum, the top midpoint of the rib cage, and marks the tips of her mastoids. He applies pressure across the base of her throat with a piece of "0" black surgical thread and uses the marking pen so that the line will last.

His physical preparation completed, Setzen looks down for the last time on Lillian Paskow's throat before he cuts it, his mind racing ahead through the procedure he has carefully planned out the night before in his study at home. He has reviewed the literature, even gone over an anatomy text. So now, ready to scrub, he is thinking, "I'll do the skin incision this way, I'll cut through the sternocleidomastoid, internal jugular, take the lymph nodes, preserve the carotid, do these moves on the larynx, suture it up this way, close."

His final preparations completed, Setzen leaves the room to scrub. When he returns, he will remove the tumor, along with the vocal cords.

When she left her hospital room forty-five minutes ago Lillian Paskow knew that she had a 75 to 80 percent chance of being cured of cancer of the larynx. She also knew, as she was being wheeled to room 1A, that she would never again speak with the voice that had been hers since infancy.

5

"I'm trying to get over the shock of what's happening to me," Lillian Paskow says, in the hoarse, scratchy rasp her speech has become. "I wake up every day and think I'm in a nightmare. What if I'm in pain and something's happening and they can't hear me? I would think everybody's afraid of that. The waiting is the most horrible thing out of all of this. It's awful."

Paskow is sitting at the kitchen table in the modest Long Island dormered Cape she has lived in since she and her husband fled the city seventeen years earlier for a better life in the suburbs. A smoker for thirty-five years, she fiddles with a coffee mug, but this morning there is no cigarette in her hand. Eight months ago, when she developed a case of "laryngitis" that hung on for about six weeks, she gave up the habit she had acquired as an eighteen-year-old Brooklyn girl attending secretarial school in Manhattan. She recalls: "Thirty-five years ago, everybody smoked. You tried it and then you just did it. I started smoking Luckies. Then I went on to Viceroys. I smoked Viceroys for years. Then about four years ago I went to a lighter cigarette, Now, because I thought it was better for me.

"If you cut my head off, I'm fine," she says, making a

weak attempt at humor. "I always had a raspy, hoarse voice. I always felt good, though, no problems," she says. "And I'm not one to call the doctor for every little thing. Not me. I have to really feel like something's wrong for me to go. And I think you know when something's really wrong."

Her laryngitis did finally drive her to a physician, who examined her throat and sent her home with a prescription for an antibiotic. But the irritation hung on through November and worried her to the point that she quit smoking, despite having an occasional smoker, her husband, in the house. Her twenty-six-year-old son, Bill, and twenty-three-year-old daughter, Mary Ann, don't smoke, she says. "They hate it," she boasts. "If the parents smoke, the kids smoke? That's baloney. They hate it. And as they were growing up they heard all this stuff about smoking being bad. When I was young, we didn't. But even when I heard it, do you think I stopped? No. It was stupidity."

After about six weeks, Paskow's sore throat finally cleared up. But around Eastertime it returned. She took the antibiotics she hadn't finished in the fall, but the medication had no effect. Again, she tried to ignore the problem, but this time she was plagued by more than simple irritation: she felt a lump in her neck. "I thought it was just a gland," she says on this July morning, referring to an obvious lump in the base of her neck. A hard lump. In part because she didn't want to find out that it might be more than a simple swollen gland, and in part because friends would tell her, "Oh, that's just a gland," Paskow delayed going to the doctor. She simply got used to the constant sore throat and "swollen gland," until, one Sunday morning, she attempted to clear some phlegm from her throat and coughed up blood. "I thought, 'My God! I'm in trouble.' Then I knew there was something more. During that week I went to another doctor, and he was the one who said, 'You have a tumor.' And he's a good doctor, too, but of course you don't believe him. He said they don't really know until they get a biopsy, but from what he could see . . . Then the next day, I was hysterical crying and I ran into my boss at the drugstore where I've worked as a checkout clerk for fifteen years—he's a pharmacist. I told him what the doctor said, and it turns out he's a very good friend with a doctor at North Shore Hospital. Well, my boss got me an appointment the next day, and then the doctor there diagnosed it as the same thing. He said, 'It's a tumor and it doesn't look good.' "

Lillian Paskow went from one specialist to another, to another. And each told her the same thing: she had cancer of the larynx and she had to have her vocal cords removed. She was devastated, and terrified, and still is. And at the same time that she has been dealing with the possibility of death and prospect of major surgery, she has been involved in planning for her son's long-scheduled August wedding. Like many patients facing a potentially fatal diagnosis, she has been bargaining. "I don't think I could have handled it any better, but I just wish it could have come up after the wedding," she says. "At the time of the wedding I'll be just about getting on my feet. Have you ever heard people who have this? Can you give me some encouragement?" she begs, a catch in her already raspy voice. "They're going to teach me to talk through the stoma. That box scares me to death. I don't ever want that. I'm young enough to learn? Have you ever heard people talk with that stoma talk?" she asks, referring to the speech she will be taught that involves the controlled belching of air through a surgically created opening, or stoma, in her lower trachea. "Does it sound normal? Would you say something's wrong?" she asks. Her eyes plead for the answer she wants to hear.

"Dr. Setzen told me what they're gonna do," she explains. "They cut all the way like this," she says, drawing a finger down one side of her neck, across the base of her throat and up the other side. "He said, 'We're gonna open the window and take it all out, and then we're gonna close it.' They try not to make it too scary. But he said that in a year's time you won't even see the scar. Everybody told me

that Setzen's patients have almost a hundred percent recovery. They're all very nice, very understanding, very
compassionate. Dr. Setzen asked me if I wanted to meet
somebody, another patient, but I said no. I might hear
something I didn't like and it might prey on my mind.

"He told me I'd be in the hospital between two and four
weeks," she continues. "He said for two weeks I can't eat,
so they have to feed me intravenously. Then, I think the
third week, you start swallowing, and if swallowing and
everything's fine, then you can come home. I think I'll be
in Intensive Care for about three days, and I think once
you're out of Intensive Care, from what I can gather, the
speech therapist comes immediately to try to get you rolling. But the main point of this whole thing is they will get
all the cancer out. And the thing with throat cancer is it's
in your throat, not in your body, and they'll get it all out
and I'm gonna have a normal, healthy life. 'Cause it is a
smoker's cancer. I never knew it, but they said alcoholics
get this too. Dr. Setzen said, 'If you smoke, or drink, I can't
do the operation.' I thought he was kidding when he said
'drink.' But I wouldn't even dare smoke. Who would think
of putting a cigarette in their mouth after this? It's very
devastating, it really is."

At this point, seven days before surgery, Lillian Paskow
seems relatively relaxed about having cancer. What has her
terrified is the thought of losing her voice. "My doctor said,
'Your voice is normally raspy and hoarse, so you won't
notice that much difference in the way you sound.' They
say that a lot of people have had this. I don't see too many.
In my drugstore, I think I saw two people. And they have
that box where they sound, like, mechanical, and that scares
the hell out of me, it really does. I just hope I can learn
that esophageal speech," which involves belching up air.
"But I'm gonna take each day as it comes. Sometimes I
want to kiss the ground, because the cancer's gonna be
gone, it's gonna go away. But it's a very trying thing, losing
your voice, no matter what, and I love to talk. I just don't

want to be like a freak, you know, I want to be able to communicate with the world again, be in my own little world again. Give me back my little world, my little job. Well, no matter what happens, at least I'll be around to see my grandchildren."

But "some days I just cry all day; other days I can just sit and talk about it all day," she says. "I had one friend who had breast cancer. Now she's trying to give me a lot of support. She's trying to tell me, 'The most frightening part of it is when you leave your house and go to the hospital that day.' But she said once you get there, everything else goes so fast, before you know it you're goin' in and . . . I'm scared to death," Lillian Paskow says, tears filling the corners of her brown eyes. "I'm afraid that I won't talk. That's scaring me to death. You know it's gonna happen, but how do you feel when you actually open your mouth and . . . how's it hit you?" she asks, pleading once more for reassurance. "I think it must be very frustrating when you talk and nothing comes out, even though you know it's going to happen, it must be traumatic, wouldn't you think so? It must be a very scary feeling—like a nightmare where you scream and nothing comes out. You say to yourself, 'How am I going to get through to people, what if something's bothering me?' But I would imagine the nurses are all aware of it, and I'm going to be monitored anywhere, I'll be in Intensive Care. You know," she adds, "if they were givin' out awards for who's frightened the most, I would win it. I'd win it. I wish I could be asleep from the minute I leave the house to when they do it, and then wake up."

6

8:21 A.M. Lillian Paskow lies in Room 1A, reduced to a
ten-inch square of exposed skin from just below her nose
to her sternum, and five inches right and left of the midline
of her throat. The Betadine antiseptic used to scrub her
skin has turned to bright yellowish brown the one island
of flesh visible in a sea of blue surgical drapes and towels.
Surgeon Michael Setzen stands to the immediate left of
Paskow's head. His partner, Philip Perlman, stands to Setz-
en's left. Chief resident Jim Sullivan, in his right hand a
Bouvie cautery with a number five needlelike blade, stands
across the table from Setzen, ready to begin. The head-
and-neck surgeon nods, and, ever so delicately, Sullivan
uses the cautery blade to trace the line Setzen has drawn.
Tiny droplets of blood ooze from the cut, and a thin haze
of gray smoke wafts upward, heavy with the stench of burning human flesh, as the electric instrument melts through
skin and the yellowish fat beneath it, sealing off blood vessels as it cuts them.

With Setzen maintaining upward pressure on the bottom
edges of the flap Sullivan has created, the chief resident
gently frees more and more of the protective covering of
Lillian Paskow's throat and neck from the layers beneath.

Now Setzen places small surgical hooks, with silk sutures attached, to the edges of the flap, and gently but firmly pulls back the flap, up over the patient's chin. He then anchors the sutures behind her head with surgical clamps. "This procedure gives you some of the nicest anatomy," Perlman tells Sullivan. "It's nice and clean and right in front of you."

In fact, at this moment, as Setzen is placing the surgical hooks, Lillian Paskow looks far more like a cadaver in an anatomy lab than she does a surgical patient. Because the electric cautery has sealed off each of the blood vessels that it has burned its way through, the scene is virtually bloodless, leaving the muscles of Paskow's neck cleanly exposed from sternum to chin, and as easily identifiable as those in an anatomy text. To an observer, what is happening on the table resembles nothing so much as one of those promotion pieces about the making of a movie: Lillian Paskow is the star, and after a long day on the set the layers of latex used to create her face are being peeled away.

Scrub nurse Kathleen Kerr, who with seven years' O.R. experience is no mere observer, draws a comparison between what she is seeing and what she reads for entertainment. "Stephen King is my favorite author," she says, adjusting the cautery power for Sullivan. "I think what I like is all the blood. In here, it's not real"—perhaps because it is the norm. "But in his books you follow the character and then he gets decapitated or something, and there's all that blood and you think, 'Ooooooooh!' That reaction makes you more human."

7

8:41 A.M. By now, work has begun in earnest in eleven of the fifteen available rooms. The case scheduled for Room 6 has been delayed by the overnight emergency, but that procedure was completed fifteen minutes ago, and a three-man cleaning crew has just begun readying the room.

This July morning is starting off as a typical day in the Main O.R. There are forty-three scheduled procedures, patients ranging in age from eight days to ninety-five years, with the average patient being fifty-seven years old. Before the day ends:

A pediatric cardiac surgeon will attempt to correct an infant's lethal heart defect; a thirty-seven-year-old man will finally have the spinal surgery he has been fearfully postponing for a year; a seventeen-year-old boy, comatose since an auto accident forty days ago, will have a gangrenous leg amputated; a sixty-year-old woman, whose father died at thirty-nine of a heart attack and whose brother died of a heart attack at thirty-seven, will have her badly deteriorated aortic valve replaced; three patients, ranging in age from fifteen to fifty-five, will undergo laparoscopic cholecystectomies—a procedure in which their gallbladders are removed using miniaturized instruments and a videocamera inserted through three tiny incisions in their abdomens; a three-month-old boy with a cleft palate and lip will enter the O.R. looking like a monster and, if all goes as planned, after the first of several plastic surgery procedures to correct his deformity will leave looking like a normal little boy; a seventeen-year-old high school athlete will have the torn tendons in her knee repaired; and colorectal surgeons will perform an abdomino-perianal resection, a bloody, disfiguring procedure, on a seventy-six-year-old man whom less radical treatment failed to cure.

On any given day it may appear as if the O.R. has been scheduled by someone with a set of dice and a grudge against surgeons and patients. And that is close to the way scheduling used to work, before 1989 when Anthony J. Tortolani took over as chairman of the Department of Surgery and instituted the "block time" system. The "block time" system involves giving each surgical specialty—cardiac, orthopedic, plastic, otolaryngology, vascular, thoracic, neuro, urological, colorectal, and general—a given amount of O.R. time on a given day, or days, each week. If surgeons in the particular specialty have not booked the time, scheduled operations, by a given deadline, then the operating time is given away to whoever needs it.

"For instance, we'll give colon and rectal surgery up to three days before to fill their block time," Tortolani explains. "If it's not filled by that group of surgeons, then we open that time to whoever has the case that we can put in there. We try to keep it in that specialty, but the time is not wasted. That's valuable real estate.

"At Glen Cove Hospital [a smaller community hospital recently absorbed by North Shore], where the physicians have a lot to say about how things run, a fellow who's been there for many years may say, 'I'm operating at eight A.M. I don't care if somebody else has a sicker patient that should go first, that's my time.' Or, 'I can't operate at two o'clock, that's office hours.' Or 'I can't operate then, that's my day off.' They can get away with that at a lot of places. But here, we say, 'Here's your time.' Sometimes a surgeon will say to me, 'I can't get my patients on the schedule, I have a sick patient.' And when I check it out, what it is is that they've offered him three or four different options, and he doesn't want to take Tuesday, because that's his office hours or he wants to take the afternoon off. He wants nine A.M. Tuesday after M and M" [the weekly Morbidity and Mortality rounds, the meeting at which case outcomes are reviewed. Surgery in the Main O.R. starts later that day]. Tortolani says that he knows that, in the past, surgeons would give tickets to Broadway shows and "special" Christmas presents to those in charge of booking the O.R.s. "I know what that's about. It's about getting prime O.R. time," Tortolani says. "What we do now is all of the staff surgeons give me the money at Christmas and all the attendings put in whatever they want—we ask for $100 a guy—and we have a big Christmas party for everybody who works in surgery. That cuts down on the 'gifts.'

"When I took over we looked at how much time each specialty was using, and every couple of months we will review who's using their time and who's not," the cardiac surgeon continues. "If somebody complains to me, 'I'm getting screwed,' we'll take a look and say, 'What do you want, what's going on?' If you don't handle it that straightforward way, it's like running a kindergarten, and I refuse to do that."

This morning, with four operations still to begin, the "lounge" serving the Main O.R. is still overflowing with nurses, technicians, surgeons, and anesthesiologists enjoying a last cup of coffee or bite of a bagel or doughnut. Pediatric cardiac surgeon Vincent Parnell and Henry So, an attending pediatric surgeon, sit talking together, jammed up against one of the two large, round tables that take up all the space in the sixteen-by-sixteen-foot room not filled by a battered couch, a decrepit end table, a refrigerator, a microwave oven, and a few storage cabinets.

Their backs are to the lounge bulletin board, to which someone has added a new message this morning:

Great deeds are usually wrought at great risks.
                                                    Herodotus 484–420 B.C.

For all of us in surgery, these are times of great risks.

Vinnie Parnell, who runs the busiest pediatric open heart surgery program—and the program with the lowest mortality rate—in New York State, is venting his frustration over a recent run-in with the Radiology Department. He tells his colleague that he called Boston Children's Hospital for a consultation on an infant with a defect that Parnell suspected was a rare congenital defect known as a "double aortic arch." To his disgust, but not surprise, Parnell was told that the Boston hospital would be "happy to take the patient"! And then they told him that the first thing they would do for the child was perform an angiogram, a test that could just as easily—and effectively—be performed at North Shore. In fact, an angiogram at North Shore confirmed Parnell's initial diagnosis, at which point a second North Shore radiologist told Parnell, "I knew at one week that that baby had a double aortic arch." "Oh? Where was it written down?" Parnell says he asked the radiologist. "I laid out the ultrasound report. I laid out all the other studies. 'Where is it written, *double aortic arch?*'

"I have to rely on them," Parnell continues, his frustration palpable. "You see something once, twice in your entire career, you have to rely on the information they give you. If they say it's a double aortic arch, I operate. If they say it's not, I don't."

"They never say, 'It is this, it is that,' " his colleague responded. "They say 'Consistent with . . .'! 'Compatible with'! Never, 'It is.' 'Consistent with . . .' That's how they're trained. 'Compatible with . . .' Never take responsibility."

B. D. Colen

"Dr. Parnell?" asks a voice emanating from a speaker mounted by the wall phone.

"Yes?"

"This is Mary. In Room 3. The nursery called and said they'll have the baby down in less than ten minutes."

"I'm on my way," Parnell says to the disembodied voice. As he pushes his chair back from the table and stands up, he turns back to So and concludes the discussion, saying, "We're trained to take responsibility. I want to know: is it a double aortic arch or isn't it?" He walks out of the lounge and down the hall toward O.R. 3, shaking his head.

8

8:56 A.M. The early morning fog has dissipated. Bright summer sunlight fights its way through the partly open blinds to flood the teenager's room. It is a small room, about twelve feet square, and it is typically adolescent: the wall opposite the foot of the bed is completely covered with photos of friends, one grouping of which is labeled *The Gang.* There is a banner for a favorite football team—the New York Jets—and there are a few risqué pinups sharing the space with photos of family trips and a large painting of the Blessed Virgin. A San Diego Chargers football cap, autographed by the members of the starting lineup, sits on the radiator beneath the window. The scene is completed by the presence of the boy's mother, a petite blond woman in a tailored suit, bending over the bed, quietly calling to her son, attempting to wake him.

Just as she has been doing, virtually all her waking hours, through the past forty days and nights.

For seventeen-year-old Andre Fogarassi's room is not really a room at all, but one of the thirty-five three-sided patient alcoves in the Intensive Care Unit, known as Five Tower. If the south wall of 508 is all teenage boy, the north wall is all high-tech medicine:

A Puritan/Bennett 7200 Series ventilator stands beside the hallway side of the bed, quietly hissing ten times a minute as it sends moisturized air, 35 percent of which is pure oxygen, through one of the two translucent blue plastic tubes that snake over the bed rail and are joined with a Y connector to the short white tube attached to Andre's green tracheostomy fitting. A Travenol Flo-Gard 2100 Enteral Pump, clamped to an IV pole beside the bed, sends a flow of high-protein nutrients through a small-gauge clear plastic tube and into a surgically implanted port leading directly into Andre's small intestine. Syringes of epinephrine and atropine, drugs used to restart the heart, are taped above the bed, immediately available if they're needed.

Andre is a small boy, and with the crew-cut-length hair that has grown back since the neurosurgeons shaved his head following the auto accident forty days ago, he looks more like twelve than seventeen. Four teenagers were riding in the car, heading to their various homes from part-time jobs, when the driver lost control and the car hit a tree. Andre's three friends were treated at a local hospital for minor bruises and bumps and sent home. Andre, whose head had hit the car's rear window, was unconscious and had to undergo emergency neurosurgery to relieve the pressure caused by bleeding within his skull. Twenty-seven days later, just when he was beginning to show the first flickers of improvement, if not consciousness, he suffered cardiac arrest and sank deeper into coma. Now, still comatose, he is also suffering from a severely gangrenous left leg, a condition caused by a blood clot in a major artery in the limb.

Andre Fogarassi is dying a piece at a time. This morning, Andre's mother and father wait for their only child to be taken to the Main O.R., where vascular surgeon Larry Scher will amputate the gangrenous leg. "You're going to do this one, it's okay, baby," Andre's mother whispers to him. "There are a lot of people pulling for you here. You've been strong before. One more time. Come on, Sweetie, you can do it." She bends further over the bed to kiss her son's pink, full cheek. His father, crying, steps back into the hallway so that a member of the hospital cleaning crew can empty the wastebasket in the alcove. Routine, after all, is routine. And Five Tower, which was opened for patients only weeks before Andre's admission to the hospital, is designed with routine—and crisis—in mind.

Unlike other areas of the hospital, where the patient is the obvious primary focus of concern for architects and interior designers, in Five Tower, as in the Main O.R., the needs of the staff come first. "In the rest of the hospital we are concerned with three factors in terms of the environment," explains Gerald Luss, North Shore's director of facilities management, a title that belies his role as the principal designer of the hospital's interior spaces. "Our first concern is the patient, two is the staff, and three is the visitor, with staff and patient being very much on the same level, and visitor being subservient to that, but still very, very important.

"But in the O.R., the patient is brought into the holding area, is prepped, and by the time they go through the doors they don't know what they're going into," Luss continues. "It's much the same in Five Tower. There, too, the important thing is the staff, much more so than the patient, because the patient is pretty much out of it. But in terms of what an environment can do to augment the psyche, the general good feeling of the staff and what they're doing, and the support of the institution, that's the most important part that environment has to play. Actually, the most important thing is the configuration of the space and of the room in support of that patient on the O.R. table or in the Intensive Care bed." Thus the open alcoves in the unit, allowing free flow of patients to and from the Main O.R.,

ease of staff and equipment around the beds, and observation of patients from the central nursing area and from
the hallway.

At this moment, for instance, Maria Sanchez sits at the
nursing station ostensibly doing paperwork but surrepti-
tiously watching the tableau in 508, directly in front of her.
The I.C.U. nurse's son is a friend of Andre's. "He's really
doing a job on us emotionally, all the nurses," she says,
quietly. "He's so young. When they're old, you expect this,
but with someone so young . . . I'm glad he's not my child.
If it was my son, I'd unplug the respirator."

9

9:07 A.M. "Feel where I am? Take your fingertip," plastic surgeon Pamela Gallagher says to the two residents assisting her in Room 5. She reaches forward and grasps the index finger of plastic surgery resident Nicholas Daniels and gently lays it on the upper lip of the cherubic brown baby lying on the operating table. "Can you feel my scissor?" Gallagher asks as she manipulates the tiny surgical instrument with her right hand. Daniels nods. "It's almost like loosening up a crumpled rug on a floor," the surgeon explains. "I'm trying to loosen it up, and hopefully, when the 'floor' is straightened, the rug will straighten out."

Three-month-old Rashid Livingston has a cleft palate, an opening in the roof of his mouth, and a cleft lip that extends all the way up into his nose. Today he is undergoing the first of a series of reconstructive operations intended to leave him looking and functioning normally. This first procedure will repair the external defect, the opening in his lip and nose, so that he will appear normal to those in the world around him. When the wounds Gallagher is now making are healed, Rashid will be fitted with a prosthesis that will fill the gap in his palate, allowing him to develop normal speech, and at about nine months he will return to the O.R. to have the palate itself repaired.

Though she has examined Rashid on a number of occasions, when she entered the O.R. at 7:40, Pam Gallagher once again meticulously mapped out the work that lay ahead of her. As anesthesiologist Jim Walsh anesthetized Rashid, who was lying on the upper end of the O.R. table, Gallagher bent over the table's lower end and used a marking pen to sketch out the planned operation on the green surgical drape covering the table's black plastic-covered mattress. "One of the big discoveries of the century is that there was more material there than surgeons thought," Gallagher told first-year-resident Roger Pitfick, referring to the flesh of the cleft lip. As she used a marking pen to draw a rough diagram of Rashid's face, she told the resident, "If you see people who had these repairs thirty years ago, there's no shape to their lip. But the most important thing in plastic surgery is to be able to see what you've got to work with."

By 8:22, after she has scrubbed and covered her blue paper pants and top with a matching paper surgical gown—one of 470, at $3 each, that the staff of the Main O.R. will use and throw away today—Gallagher begins marking her small patient's face with the sharpened end of a cotton swab stick and a purple dye. Her latex-gloved hands glowing white in the bright surgical lights, she makes a series of tiny dots along the infant's upper lip and nose, marking the path she will follow with scalpel and scissors. But after stepping back for a moment to survey her work, she announces to the residents that she's not happy with her dots and asks for an eraser. "Eighty percent of this operation is the markings," she explains. "If you screw up your dots, then you don't have your landmarks. If you err on narrowness, then you can't repair it. But if we err in fullness, we can fix it."

Viewed from his left side, Rashid Livingston looks normal as he lies on his back. He is, in fact, a beautiful child, a brown-skinned Renaissance cherub. But on closer examination, it is obvious that three-quarters of the tissue that is his nose and upper lip is on the left side of his facial midline, while only a quarter sits on the fissure that runs from his open mouth up the right side of his nose. So Gallagher uses her sharpened stick and ink to draw a new midline for nose and lip, and then, having completed the markings on the left side of the face, she tells the residents: "The rest of this is all fudge factor. One of the crappiest things I've seen in repairs is the destruction of the wing, from here to here." She points from the right corner of Rashid's mouth to the end of the apparent lip.

Pam Gallagher's next step in the reconstruction of Rashid Livingston's face is to make a template with a piece of Steri-strip. She then takes a 25-gauge needle and her purple dye and, guided by the template, "tattoos" a dotted line, creates the line her scalpel will follow along Rashid's face.

10

9:08 A.M. "Dr. Walker? Can I speak with you a minute? We've got a little problem."

"Sure. What have you got?" Peter Walker, chairman of the Department of Anesthesia, asks Main O.R. head nurse Diana Potenza. Walker has finished his work on the emergency in Room 6 and spent 30 minutes in the Anesthesia Department office going over the day's schedule. Now he is about to begin his previously scheduled case, when Potenza catches up with him near the nursing station.

As Potenza and Walker lean against the wall near the entrance to the Main O.R., the head nurse complains that the Anesthesia Department, which is really a private practice group, is refusing to let surgical residents use its bronchoscope, the fiber-optic instrument used to visualize the vocal cords and main tubes of the lungs. While she has nothing to do with the training or scheduling of the residents, she is directly responsible for the daily running of the operating rooms, and thus finds herself interceding on behalf of the surgical trainees. She points out that last night the senior resident on call needed to use a scope and the anesthesiologist on call wouldn't let the resident use Anesthesia's instrument. Walker, who serves as the intermediary between the group of 37 anesthesiologists and other hospital departments, such as Nursing, Surgery, and Administration, backs up Anesthesia. It's up to the Department of Surgery to supply a bronchoscope for the residents, he tells Potenza. Though conducted in muted tones, the "discussion" sounds like a kindergarten argument about sharing a red wagon, which is out of character for both Potenza, whose job is to grease the Main O.R.'s wheels, and Walker, who is, at least on the surface, its Henry Clay. Until, that is, it becomes apparent that the argument is really about money, and a not insubstantial amount of it. Walker points out that, as a theoretically independent group of practitioners, the anesthesiologists have to purchase their own bronchoscope; the hospital does not supply it.

"But Dr. Walker, the residents need it," Potenza politely insists.

Walker, a soft-spoken administrator whose manner could almost be described as courtly, is not about to compromise this time. "Talk to Dr. Tortolani about having the Department of Surgery get one. We're on our fourth bronchoscope—at $7,000 a pop—so if you think I'm being sensitive, you're right," he says, ending the conversation and slapping his hand against the pressure switch plate that causes the doors to the central hallway of the Main O.R. to swing open.

Diana Potenza returns to her tiny office on the periphery of the Main O.R. and makes a note to call chief of surgery Anthony J. Tortolani.

11

Diana Potenza and Tony Tortolani go back a long way together, to the summer of 1976, when she was a young assistant head nurse in the cardiac surgery program at New York University Medical Center, and he was a young surgeon just beginning his fellowship in cardiac surgery. At that point, Potenza was five years out of Wesley College, in Dover, Delaware, where she had earned her associate degree in nursing. Following graduation, she and a friend had left Dover for NYU, where they were hoping to land jobs in I.C.U. nursing. "I went directly into the Operating Room," she recalls, sitting in the living room of her home, a five-minute drive from North Shore and the Main O.R.

"I wanted to go into the I.C.U. I liked the monitors, I liked the sick patients, I liked that type of pace. NYU didn't have any openings in the I.C.U., only openings in the Operating Room. But we took a chance—and we stayed for five years. I went through all of the specialty areas there, and then for the last two years I was in cardiac."

Potenza's tenure at NYU ended in December 1976, just five months after Tortolani began his two years there. The daughter of an itinerant school superintendent, Diana Potenza had never lived more than three years in one place while she was growing up, and moving on was as much a part of her nature as a driving desire to move up. So having spent two years under Dr. Frank Spencer, one of East Coast heart surgery's living legends, she applied for and got a job in California, in Dr. Norman Shumway's world-renowned heart transplantation program at Stanford University Medical Center, in Palo Alto.

"It was wonderful and exciting. I found a whole different philosophy in medicine, coming from the East and going to the West. When they say 'laid-back' in the West, they really mean it. The first month or so I used to make them very nervous," says Potenza, a small, intense woman with constantly probing blue eyes. "I would get everything done in the first forty-five minutes of a case, always preparing for an emergency. Everybody else sort of took their time —they got things done, but not in the manner that I did. I was very fast and it made them nervous until they got used to my style. And I calmed down also, slowed down. When an emergency occurred, everybody was very calm and just did things. You didn't even know there was a real problem: you just went and did things. There was no yelling or screaming, it was very well organized, very well directed, everybody knew what to do, somebody just took charge of the surgical aspect, somebody took charge of the anesthesia, even from the nursing aspect. I was very impressed. It was a very nice atmosphere to work in. People spoke nicely to people and they weren't back-stabbing."

Potenza worked at Stanford for two years, when Norman Shumway had one of the world's few successful heart transplant programs. But by 1978, the combination of wanderlust and need for career movement had her looking around again. She had been doing extra work as a registry nurse, filling in at other area hospitals, and thus heard about an opening as an assistant head nurse in cardiac surgery at the University of California at San Francisco. That, Potenza decided, was the job for her, because it would mean a chance to get experience under Dr. Paul Ebert, one of the

leading lights in pediatric cardiac surgery. So she spent the
next two years working in Ebert's program, learning management skills that would stand her in good stead throughout her career.

In 1980, Potenza ran into Tony Tortolani at one of the
major cardiac surgery meetings. He told her that he had
recently begun practice at North Shore, and along with his
partner, Michael Hall, was attempting to fashion a first-
class cardiac surgery program at the community hospital.
Remembering Potenza's efficiency from their days together
at NYU, Tortolani asked her if she would be interested in
building up the nursing component of his fledgling program.

Diana Potenza looked the hospital over and decided that
the job offered a wonderful opportunity for her to grow
and develop, because not only was it a position in which
she could hone the management skills she had developed
at U.C. San Francisco, but also it offered a rare chance to
develop a program from scratch. "I took something that
was not very well organized and I got to grow into it and
develop it the way that I wanted to do it. I was the boss. I
made the decisions. I trained the staff. It was really a lot
of fun. They had a team of nurses, but they didn't really
have any leadership there. Nobody had ever worked anywhere else, had ever gone to any other program, they were
trained at North Shore, they really never went to any other
hospitals to see how they were doing it. And here were two
young guys that wanted to develop the cardiac program,
but they knew nothing about the nursing aspects of de-
veloping it and they needed somebody to work on that for
them while they were getting patients and perfecting their
skills and techniques to build up a good reputation for
themselves."

Working on the East Coast again was a shock to Potenza's
professional system, "after working in California, where
everything was modern technology and they were up on
the latest trends in nursing. The East is not as innova-

tive, I don't care where you are: New York, Boston. They weren't at North Shore at the time," she says. "They were just beginning to realize that they had to make changes, and slowly and surely the changes were made. Cardiac surgery was the first step in making those changes for the Operating Room. It was fun for me because I was there, I saw the way it was when I first came here and I was a part of all this change. We developed a team, we brought in disposables, I developed the philosophy and the practice of sterile instrumentation for all the specialty areas, specialty sets for the specialty areas." She explains, "Prior to that they had basic trays and added instruments. They didn't have designated sets. So we developed all the specialty sets and it was a long process, and an expensive process, but the busier they got in the Operating Room, the more important it was."

With a staff of 100 registered nurses and 50 licensed practical nurses, O.R. techs, monitor techs, unit aides, and transporters, who bring patients to the Main O.R. from their rooms, scheduling is one of Potenza's biggest headaches. The main day nursing shift runs from 7:00 A.M. to 3:00 P.M., with 28 to 30 RNs working those hours. Additionally, on any given day, there are two to three nurses on a 9 to 5 shift, three to four on an 11:15 A.M. to 7:15 P.M. schedule, eight nurses who work from 2:45 in the afternoon until 10:15 at night, and four who work the overnight shift, from 11:00 P.M. to 7:00 A.M. The way the system is designed, there are ten to fifteen day shift nurses still working their regular hours at 3:00 P.M., when each day four or five of the early shift nurses who are scheduled to leave are kept on on overtime. Thus, with all the varying shifts and overtime, Potenza ends up with 22 to 26 nurses who are still on until 7 P.M., when the O.R. day theoretically ends, and another eight or nine nurses who are still on until 11:00 P.M. "Only the cardiac staff is officially on call, and that's two people to do cardiac cases only. We have four people on, so we can run two rooms for emergencies after 11 o'clock. If they have to open a third room, they would go through the list to get somebody who could come in, or the evening staff would stay if the case was already in progress."

Tortolani says that he has basically given Diana Potenza a free hand in running the Main O.R., telling her that she makes the rules and he will abide by them and see that all the staff and attending surgeons do likewise. Told that she is credited by some with setting the tone for the O.R., Potenza responds: "If the tone is good, that's a nice compliment. If the tone is bad . . .

"I try to promote professionalism between the nurses and the residents—we had a lot of problems with the residents not cooperating, not being professional. I met with the chief residents. I met with Dr. Tortolani. The staff and attending physicians [community-based surgeons with O.R. privileges at North Shore] set the tone for the residency program. If they're professional to the nurses, then they set the tone for the third-year residents, and the second-years and the first-years will learn to act that way. I don't like people that don't work together and who aren't professional. We had problems with the way people spoke to each other, whether it was attending-to-attending, attending-to-the-anesthesiologists, attending-to-the-residents, attending-to-the-nurses. I wouldn't tolerate attendings being unprofessional with the nurses. I will confront them. I'll confront them at the time, I'll confront them afterward. I had some roundabout discussions with a lot of them about the way they acted unprofessional. The coordinator at the front desk probably gets the most verbal abuse of anybody in the Operating Room. A case gets pushed back an hour and a half and then that pushes back the next surgeon an hour and a half and he has office hours, and then he gets frustrated. But what I find with the attendings is that they will not confront each other. They will not say to their colleague, 'I can't believe you took this long, I'm delayed, I'm really upset, you came late, why did you come in late?' But they will verbally abuse the coordinator at the front desk, or the secretaries at the front desk: it's much easier than confronting their colleague." Potenza says she will try to work with the surgeons, explaining the problem to them and asking for their cooperation. But if she doesn't get it, she has no hesitation about reporting the problem to the chairman of their subspecialty department and to Tony Tortolani, who will leave the problem to the department chiefs—unless they fail to deal with it. "I've been in the job almost two years now, and it took six or seven months for the surgeons and the residents to realize that I'm not here to be a bad guy or to get them into trouble. I'm here to make them professionals and to help them understand that working together is important, because the more you work together, the better the flow of the day is," Potenza explains. "They realize now that they can't act out like that. Medicine is a business now. It's not like the surgeon is the almighty God, or the anesthesiologist is the almighty God, and when they speak, everyone bows down to them.

"Sometimes the surgeons get upset and crazy at the situation that's happening. The patient may go bad at a certain time, and they get excited and yell," Potenza says. "And then everything's under control and everything's okay again. Those things happen in the Operating Room and if you're going to work in the Operating Room, you have to realize that too, and you have to be able to overlook a situation like that and you have to be able to handle it yourself emotionally when things get bad and tense. And when it's over with, it's over with, and nobody's meant any harm by it. But some people are just abusive people; they're nasty." When that happens, Potenza will quietly take a surgeon aside and say, "There are a lot of nurses that do not like to work with you because of your behavior, and this can't be tolerated in the Operating Room." In other words, shape up, Buddy, or you're going to be functioning as your own scrub nurse and circulating nurse. "In general," Potenza adds, "most of the surgeons are very nice to work with. You have a few who are very condescending, and that's just their personality, and you can't do anything about it. And I tell the nurses, 'That's their personality, we can't change their personality, but they have no right to verbally abuse you on anything, for any reason at all.' I always tell the nurses, 'Let me know, and I will speak to them, I'll take it to the proper personnel.' So they come to me."

Despite the common image of the surgeon as an ego-maniac, heaping abuse on nurses and flinging instruments around the O.R. when things aren't going as he thinks they should, Potenza says, "Most of the surgeons work quite well with the nurses. We only have four or five who cause problems. One of the vascular surgeons tends to scream and yell a lot. One of the general surgeons tends to be nasty and condescending. And we have a plastic surgeon who's that way, who the nurses don't like to work with. We used to have another plastic surgeon who verbally abused the patients. He did a lot of patients under local and he'd yell at them: 'Don't move! You're going to screw it up!' I couldn't figure out why anyone would go to him. To be yelled at by your surgeon?"

Being an O.R. head nurse is the hospital equivalent of being an air traffic controller. With 15 cases in progress and two dozen other surgeons and patients waiting to go, Potenza and her two assistant head nurses are constantly monitoring the progress of the various cases to gauge what is happening to the day's schedule and see where more staff may be needed. The biggest disaster she can face, she says, is to have all the rooms full and then "have a trauma in the Emergency Room that needs to come up, and so we don't have an operating room available," she explains. "Say you have a gunshot wound to the heart, a stab wound to the heart, a motor vehicle accident, or you have a cardiac patient who crashes in the cath lab and has to come up right away for an emergency bypass. That's the worst thing that can happen to you—and it happens every couple of months. What we do is make rounds in the back—[which is how the staff refers to the area of the Main O.R. taken up by the operating rooms]—to find out which room is coming out first, and that's the room that we put that emergency in. Sometimes the emergency has to wait 30, 45 minutes, before something is ready to break. But whatever room breaks first is the room that we'll put that emergency in. But we don't have the luxury to keep an operating room open for any type of an emergency, because we're limited with our operating rooms as it is, and we have such an overabundance of cases that need to get done that we can't leave a room open for emergencies."

Similar strains in the O.R. schedule result when a trauma case is still going from the night before, as is the case today. "All the cases scheduled for that room for the day get delayed," Potenza says. At that point, all the surgeons with scheduled cases in the affected room have to be notified of the delay and told that they'll be called later in the day with new operating times. Similarly, the day's schedule may be thrown off when a busy night has resulted in unexpected admissions to the Surgical Intensive Care Unit. Then those cases that will obviously need I.C.U. beds after surgery are delayed until surgeons can make rounds and determine who, if anyone, can be moved out of the I.C.U. to free beds.

While all of this makes Potenza's job one that an observer would describe as "high pressure," she insists she doesn't feel it. "Somebody else might, but I don't take it to heart," she says. "When problems arise, I'm a crisis manager. You read all the books saying 'plan out your time and plan your day.' Well, it's very difficult when you work in an operating room to really plan everything out. I have an agenda of what needs to be accomplished in that day, and I get as much done as I can, but there's so much crisis management that you do what you can continuously throughout the day. Then as a situation arises, you handle it, you take care of it. Another situation arises, you handle it, you take care of it. I don't dwell on it. I don't take it home with me. Once it's over and it's done with, as far as I'm concerned it's over and done with. I may take it to the proper personnel, I might follow up on it, but I don't dwell on it. If I dwelt on it, I wouldn't be in the position. Sometimes I'm convinced you really have to have a degree in psychiatry to do this."

And Diana Potenza could probably use psychiatric expertise to deal with the pressures of 12 hours a day in the Main O.R. and a home life that includes a three-year-old son, three stepchildren, ranging in age from nine to twenty—all of whom live with her and her husband, Joe —a cat, a nearly blind dog, and a live-in housekeeper. Her husband, who is a regional vice president of one of the world's largest medical supply businesses, understands what she's dealing with at work, and has been able to provide her with advice and emotional support, she says. "He's like me, he doesn't get crazy either." But the person she considers her "real lifesaver is Madge, who is my housekeeper, who keeps everything under control and enables me to work." Potenza explains: "She came the week after Matthew was born and she's been here since. That's what keeps me from being crazy. I don't have to worry about picking children up at a babysitter. I go to work at six-thirty in the morning, and sometimes I don't get home till six or seven if it's a busy, crazy day. Sometimes I go back in the evening, too."

The O.R., Potenza says, is "the unknown place" to anyone who doesn't work there. "When you work in the Operating Room, you have to be specially trained to work there. You cannot just take any nurse and put her in the Operating Room and have her function. It's a highly technical, different type of nursing skill that you learn, dealing with the needs of the patient. You're the patient advocate. The patient's only awake in the Operating Room for maybe 15 or 20 minutes and it's your total responsibility to make sure that the patient is positioned properly, that it's a safe environment for the patient, that it's a sterile environment, you're monitoring everything with that patient. Anesthesia is in control of one aspect of their care, but you're in control of everything else. The surgeon does the surgical procedure on the patient, but you're making sure that everything is flowing, that sterile technique is being maintained, that all the counts [of instruments, needles, gauze pads, and all other disposables] are done properly and they're all correct.

"It's also not something that you can learn in a week or two. Our orientation program, for somebody who doesn't know anything about O.R. nursing, is six months. After you're finished with that, you're able to function on your own, but it's a couple of years before you're really comfortable working in the Operating Room and feel that you can rotate through services and be able to function well. And it just comes from working in the Operating Room and handling the different situations. You're always in the Operating Room, you never work anywhere else."

Despite the need for intensive training and specialization, to say nothing of increased responsibility, the pay scale for nurses in the Main O.R. is the same as that for nurses everywhere else in the hospital: a nurse with twenty-five years' experience, at the top of the scale, can make $50,000 a year, plus overtime. "The problem with nursing is there's nowhere to go," Potenza says. "The salaries don't increase. Even if you have your Ph.D., there's no way you're making $200,000 a year. A top salary for a director of nursing is $80,000 to maybe around $100,000—tops." Potenza feels quite strongly that nurses, as a professional group, missed a luxury liner when it sailed about ten to fifteen years ago. "Nursing forced the medical profession into creating the physician's assistant program, which really should have been a higher scale job for nurses to go into. The problem with nursing is they've really defeated themselves, instead of working together. I think it has to do with it being a profession with a majority of women. Women don't have that team concept. I think it stems from childhood, not playing team sports, where in the male-dominated world, a lot of them played team sports, they're used to working together and not fighting. That's why I enjoyed working in the cardiac department. I was working with all the men, myself and my staff. They were very supportive, they don't get crazy about things."

Potenza insists: "There's a lot of cutthroat stuff with a lot of nurses. It's pettiness. If they forgot about the little stuff and worked together to follow the policy and procedure and make sure everybody's working together, you wouldn't have these small little problems: they don't like the way this one speaks to them, or I get the problems: 'My scrub nurse always goes out and has coffee and I have to do the room myself.' 'Why are you letting her go out there? Why don't you tell her? Give her directions, go do this, go do that.' They'd rather come to me and complain about it than confront their peers with it," she says, describing the same behavior she complains of in surgeons, all but three of whom at North Shore are male.

12

9:14 A.M. "I'll be the most amazed person in the world if they have this baby down in ten minutes. It usually takes them twenty minutes just to wrap it up and send it down here," Vinnie Parnell remarks to Peter Walker. But no sooner do the words reverberate off Room 3's tile walls than a nurse from the Intensive Care Nursery pushes open the light brown wooden door with her rear end and pulls a transport isolette into the room. "For Baby Morrell to O.R. 8 A.M." reads a hand-lettered card on the clear plastic box used to transport infants.

In the O.R. scheduled times are relative, more useful for predicting the order of events than the precise moment they will occur. Thus it is safe to assume that the operation scheduled to begin at 11:30 in O.R. 12 will begin after the procedure scheduled for 7:30, and before that planned for 1:30. It is never safe to assume, however, that any of those cases will begin at the times scheduled, because any delay in the ending of the previous case, a late arrival on the part of the surgeon—who might be held up on rounds, or seeing patients in the office—any difficulty in anesthetizing the patient, or a shortage of transporters to bring the patients to the Main O.R., any of these factors can defer the start of surgery. And inevitably will. It is 9:14 A.M., and while the hallways are crowded with personnel, equipment, and four patients on gurneys waiting to be moved into operating rooms, and while nurses and technicians are preparing rooms for patients, four of the scheduled morning cases have yet to get under way. Parnell is, after all, startled to see his patient arrive now, despite the fact that he had a scheduled start time of 8:30.

By now, perfusionist Bridget Lindstrom, who runs the heart-lung machine, or "pump," and nurses Mary Brian and Denise Coletti have completed their initial preparations for the open heart surgery scheduled for eight-day-old David Joseph Morrell. The two nurses, working to the left and at the bottom of the operating table, have draped instrument stands and laid out sterile instruments and supplies. More than 150 stainless steel scissors, clamps, spreaders, needle holders—three with needles and sutures already clamped in their jaws—are already laid out, along with fifty sutures in different shapes and sizes and dozens of the cotton pads called sponges. In this twenty-four-hour period, the work in the Main O.R. will call for the consumption of 1,000 packs of sutures, each containing between one and ten needles, in a myriad of shapes and sizes, with sutures attached. The surgeons and O.R. staff will also go through 5,000 surgical sponges, 120 drapes, 500 pairs of latex gloves, 470 gowns, 80 surgical staple guns, 47 endotracheal tubes, and 700 masks. And every one of those 7,917 items will end up in a trash can—and most will be on some patient's bill.

Denise Coletti is scrubbing for this case, which means she will remain in the sterile area, preparing sutures and passing equipment to the surgeons as requested. Mary Brian will be circulating, which makes her responsible for resupplying the instrument stands, keeping the nursing notes of the procedure, overseeing the final counts of all disposables used during the operation, and writing up charge slips for them. The relationship between surgeon and circulating nurse is not unlike that of an admiral and the captain who commands the admiral's flagship: the circulating nurse is the individual responsible for the smooth functioning of the room in which the surgeon operates, just as the captain is the officer directly in charge of the vessel from which the admiral commands his fleet.

As the nurses make their final preparations, Bridget Lindstrom is methodically checking over the pump, the machine that will make it possible for Parnell to even attempt to save the infant's life. She has already attached the disposable blood and fluid filters and clear plastic lines and valves that are replaced after each case. The twenty-four-year-old perfusionist, for whom the ultimate disaster would be to pump air into the patient's circulatory system, is checking over all the tubing for any kinks or imperfect connections.

Mary Brian lifts the alert, curious, blue-eyed infant, dressed in a disposable diaper decorated with Disney characters, out of the isolette and places him in the middle of the top third of the O.R. table. As he lies on his back, staring at the twelve Skytron lights above him, the infant's additional, external, congenital defect is shockingly apparent: in addition to the malformation of his heart, he has such a severe cleft palate and lip, extending into his nose, that his mouth appears to be a square hole in the center of his face. The nursing notes that are part of Baby Morrell's already voluminous chart state that this morning he weighs 3905 grams—8.6 pounds—and has been "cleared for O.R." At 7:15 A.M. his primary care nurse had made the observation that "parents at bedside this a.m." Her final note: "Medicated as ordered. Left N.I.C.U. at 0903."

Peter Fitz-Randolph Walker, graduate of Harvard College and Boston University Medical School, did an internship and residency in surgery at Boston's Peter Bent Brigham Hospital. Then, after serving two years as a naval surgeon, he realized he was working at the wrong end of the operating table—his was not a surgeon's ego—and he returned to Harvard to do a residency in anesthesia at Massachusetts General Hospital, followed by a fellowship in pediatric cardiac anesthesia. This is not a mere "gas passer" who is now taping five electrocardiogram leads in place on tiny David Morrell's body. "We'll have to work a little harder than we normally do to secure this tube," he says, the infant endotracheal tube in hand, "because we don't have a nostril to secure it to." He then rubs a substance called Mastisol around the infant's mouth, explaining that it's similar to the pine tar rubbed on baseball bats to improve the grip. Walker places an infant-sized face mask over the hole that is the child's nose and mouth and puts him to sleep using halothane. He is very gentle with the infant, as he is with all children. The baby is too young to need the kind of bedtime story the anesthesiologist uses with older children, but Walker extends himself in the same way. The genetic father of four and adoptive father of twin teenage girls, Peter Walker never tells a child he is putting him to sleep. "You can get anyone off to sleep," he says. "That's what veterinarians do. Oddly enough, that's one of the more unfortunate terms used around the specialty and it's one that we're trained to avoid, particularly those of us who care for children. Because all they've heard about is old Spot, who went to the vet and was 'put to sleep'— and suddenly Spot wasn't around anymore."

13

9:52 A.M. "This thing's going exceedingly well," Dr. Michael Setzen says as he clamps off a branch of Lillian Paskow's left internal jugular vein, tying it in two places before chief resident Jim Sullivan slices through it with the electric cautery. "This is a big, hard, worrisome lymph node," Setzen says, pointing to a pea-size lump in the tissue of the neck. "It should be impossible to see," he notes, explaining that the lymph nodes in the fifty-three-year-old woman's neck will be removed along with the larynx, a portion of the muscle structure, and the left internal jugular.

A surgeon working with a resident has a few basic choices to make: whether to have the resident merely observe or actively participate; and, if the resident is to participate, whether to have the resident primarily maneuver clamps and expose tissue for the surgeon or to reverse those roles. Setzen has chosen the latter options.

"Because he's a chief resident," Setzen explains, "Jim is getting to do a lot, but as long as I'm watching, it's okay. That's the concept that the public may not understand, that if the chief resident is doing some of the work, it's okay as long as he's doing it step by step under the guidance of a trained surgeon. But the surgeon is basically orchestrating the operation, not the resident. You need two people to do it, so if the surgeon is more comfortable letting the resident do some of the surgery, that's okay, because he may be better helping the resident than the resident helping him. I'm "doing" everything: I'm separating the tissues, I'm pulling up and stopping off the blood vessels, I'm tying off. All the resident is doing is cutting the tissue, which means nothing. I'm making sure the scalpel is in the right place, which he couldn't do. I'm assisting him—he couldn't assist me. He wouldn't be able to separate everything the way I can for him. He doesn't know all the moves.

"Now, we're moving to the internal jugular," he notes. "I'm saying where we're going. Cutting the tissue is really nothing. It's the steps and exposing the tissue planes that matter."

Despite having been in practice for a decade, Setzen spends the evening before planning in detail for an operation such as Paskow's.

"No matter how skilled you are, this kind of case is probably the most significant type of surgical procedure that I would do in my specialty," the otolaryngologist says. "However good I am, I'm still thinking about it the night before. I might spend a couple of hours preparing, reviewing the literature, reviewing the anatomy, thinking about the patient, thinking about my incision, thinking about the steps I might take during the procedure, and then, when I come in here in the morning, I'm going to feel a lot more comfortable. I wouldn't want that planning and reviewing going on in my mind now. I want to think about it the night before, or even days before with this kind of complicated procedure. When we come in here, I think a lot of adrenaline's pumping. We're ready to go. We've got a big procedure ahead of us, a lot of delicate and complex surgery, and someone's life is in our hands. I do a lot of simpler surgery, like tonsillectomies, sinus surgery, that's a lot easier and doesn't demand the kind of thought processing that this kind of major procedure demands.

"Once we start, our hearts are really pumping, we know we've got a lot of work ahead of us, and probably a lot of tension and anxiety. As we make our incision and ease into the case, a lot of the tension dissipates and we feel a lot more comfortable."

But looking at Lillian Paskow, lying on the operating table with all the major internal structures of her throat and neck exposed—and a good hunk of them about to be removed—doesn't a surgeon ever look down and hesitate, if only for a second, thinking, "Omigod! What am I doing here?"

Setzen says he doesn't, but on a very major case like this he may say to himself, "I've got a major job ahead of me, and am I going to be able to accomplish what I want and the patient wants? I know I can. But some of it goes through my mind and I know it goes through the resident's mind. He's there helping me, but he's not quite sure what we're going to do, and as things progress he sees this tremendous wound, and he may be saying to himself, 'Are we going to be able to close this and put her back together? We've taken everything out, are we going to be able to close her and let her leave the operating room and leave this hospital?' I think a lot of that may go through his mind." Sullivan laughs, and Setzen continues: "The things that are going through my mind are, 'Are we going to be able to get the tumor out? Are we going to be able to preserve the major vessels, mainly the carotids? Am I going to prevent this lady from getting a stroke?' I'm concerned about all the complications, and there are a multitude of them, and they're going through my mind during the entire case. I'm working with a chief resident and I've got to rely on his competence and hope that he doesn't cause me any problems, because ultimately the responsibility's going to be mine. And I have this responsibility to the patient and I don't want any complications. She and I discussed each and every complication ahead of time, but I don't want any of them to occur. If they do occur, I'll have to accept them, she'll have to accept them, this is part of our arrangement, but I'd rather come out of there complication-free with a happy patient."

At 10:01 A.M. Jim Sullivan slices free the first area of cancerous growth in Lillian Paskow's neck. In color, shape, and size it resembles nothing so much as a chicken liver. Other than the fact that it is ugly, this little bit of tissue gives no outward hint that in its uncontrolled growth it possesses the power to take over and kill the 147-pound woman in whom it has been growing.

14

10:05 A.M. Jack Hannan is terrified.

He is lying on his back on a gurney in the hallway outside the door to O.R. 12, one of the two twenty-by-twenty-five-foot rooms principally used for neurosurgery cases. He is staring at the dim fluorescent ceiling light above him, his neck held motionless in a cervical collar. "I knew this had to be done," says the thirty-seven-year-old accountant, "but with each test, the anticipation gets worse. And let me tell you, the tests suck."

Hannan had been experiencing recurrent neck aches for about a dozen years. He basically ignored the problem, other than to occasionally visit a chiropractor friend who would give him some temporary relief. But about a month ago, while lying in bed early one morning, he felt a sudden twinge and couldn't move. The chiropractor made a house call and had the good sense not to attempt manipulation this time. Hannan then went to a friend who does MRIs —magnetic resonance imaging, a noninvasive, nonradioactive imaging technique that with the aid of a computer produces detailed images of soft tissue. "He looked at the pictures and said, "Jack, you win! Surgery time. You've got herniated disks at C-6 and C-7," the bottom two vertebrae in the neck, which sit just about at the level of the shoulders.

So today Hannan lies in the hallway of the Main O.R., cringing and moaning as anesthesiologist Fred Fabiano injects his wrist with lidocaine—a local anesthetic that does burn, but usually doesn't cause moaning and writhing—before placing a larger catheter in the top of the wrist.

"You anxious?" inquires Ph.D. physiologist Joe Danto.

"Yes," Hannan hisses through clenched teeth.

"Thank God one of us is," quips Danto, a fixture in O.R. 12 when neurosurgeon Nancy Epstein is operating. Over the past several years, Danto and Epstein have together developed a still-experimental procedure to limit, if not eliminate, the nerve damage that may be caused by the cervical laminectomy procedure, the operation to remove herniated cervical disks. Danto will place wire leads on Hannan's head and hands, allowing Danto to measure "evoked potentials," the amount of time, in milliseconds, that it takes nerve impulses to travel from the hands through the area of the spine on which Epstein operates, to the brain. By measuring the times before the procedure begins, Danto can pick up on changes as the surgeon works, and he can warn her to stop if she starts to interfere with the impulses. At the end of the operation he is often able to see an immediate improvement in the response times, compared to the times prior to surgery, which tells Epstein that she has relieved pressure on the nerves and has not caused any damage while operating.

"I don't want to feel any pain," mumbles the patient, who is definitely becoming groggy.

"No pain?" Fabiano responds. "You want an incision, don't you?" He doesn't wait for a response, and, as he injects Versed into the catheter in Hannan's wrist, reassures him that he won't remember a thing. The anesthesiologist then heavily coats a small rubber nasogastric tube with a lidocaine cream and slides it into Hannan's nose and down into the back of his throat.

"It hurts," Hannan cries, weakly. "Oooo, it hurts."

"Pay his bill last," Danto jokes. Staff members standing outside of Hannan's limited field of vision roll their eyes. On a scale of 1 to 10, they say this patient rates a 9.5 for intolerance to pain and the level of his complaining. Fred Fabiano slides the greasy rubber tube out of Hannan's nostril and inserts a second, slightly larger tube. Because the patient's injury is in his neck, it will be necessary to insert the endotracheal tube for anesthesia in his throat while he is awake, without moving his neck. Fabiano uses the set of progressively larger rubber tubes to dilate the nostril until he can insert a bronchoscope with an endotracheal tube fitted over it. Using the fiber-optic bronchoscope, Fabiano will be able to see the vocal cords and guide the scope and endotracheal tube past the cords without damaging them. Then he will pull out the bronchoscope and leave the endotracheal tube in place in the trachea.

Now Danto goes to work, sticking two electrical leads on Hannan's forehead and one on top of his head. "This may look like inhuman torture," he tells the patient, "but since we've done this we've had no neurological deficits."

"Ooo! Don't pull my hair out," the patient complains, without appearing to really know what he is saying. The narcotics and the Versed he's been given have taken effect.

"Oh, you're out to lunch now, aren't you?" Danto asks, not expecting a response.

"He's on a different planet," quips Fabiano, holding open the door to Room 12 so that Hannan can be wheeled in, twenty-five minutes after receiving the initial lidocaine injection.

15

10:35 A.M. "Place the towel right at the groin and scrub to the chin," Vinnie Parnell tells Mary Brian. The circulating nurse lays a blue cotton O.R. towel across Baby Morrell's groin and then takes a plastic bottle of Betadine and squeezes the gelatinous substance all over the infant's abdomen and chest. Using a disposable sponge, she rubs the Betadine all over the exposed skin, leaving it as germ free as skin will ever be, and looking as though someone has been using soy sauce to fingerpaint on little David's body. Brian then places surgical drapes in such a way that the infant is reduced to a rectangle of exposed skin from navel to throat. Anesthesiologist Peter Walker has already placed ointment in the baby's eyes to keep them moisturized, and he has taped them shut to protect them during the hours of surgery. He then places a surgical towel over the baby's face and hangs the ether barrier—a dated misnomer, as ether isn't used in modern O.R.s, having long ago been replaced by nonflammable gases and narcotics—and the team is ready to begin work in earnest.

Using the Bovie electric cautery, Vinnie Parnell makes his initial incision, a straight, thin, vertical four-inch cut down the midline of the infant's chest. The blade, sizzling as it slices through the skin and fat, is almost instantly at the sternum. Then Parnell uses a sternal saw to cut through the sternum and split the rib cage in two. Parnell and Dominic DiCapua, a surgeon's assistant who works for the cardiac surgery group, next use a set of stainless steel chest spreaders—so small as to resemble a scale model of those used in adult surgery—to crank open the rib cage and create a work area in the chest.

"It's what Hellerstein in radiology predicted," says Parnell, looking down at David Morrell's heart after opening the pericardium, the protective membrane that surrounds the organ. "I can't really say at a conference that I don't depend upon what they predict radiographically. But radiology is right just enough for it to be a pain in the ass, right, Dom?"

"Right. And after surgery they're right one hundred percent of the time," the surgeon's assistant, says, laughing. " 'Oh yeah, that's what I saw.' "

"Well, what we see here is the aorta connected to the right ventricle, and the pulmonary artery connected to the left ventricle," Parnell says, looking down at David Morrell's deformed heart. "What we want to end up with is the aorta connected to the left ventricle, and the pulmonary artery connected to the right ventricle."

What Parnell sees on the table beneath his hands is what the radiologists told him he would find—a case of transposition of the great vessels, one of the most serious, if not the most serious, congenital heart defects that it is possible to correct. Normally, blood returning from the body enters the right atrium through the vena cava and is pumped into the right ventricle, which contracts and sends the blood out the pulmonary artery to the lungs. The blood is oxygenated in the lungs, returns to the left atrium through the pulmonary veins, and travels into the left ventricle, where it is pumped out the aorta to circulate throughout the body.

But in an infant born with transposition of the great

vessels, the oxygen-depleted blood returns to the right side of the heart, only to be pumped back to the body through the misconnected aorta. Similarly, the oxygenated blood returns from the lungs to the left side of the heart, where it is pumped back to the lungs through the misplaced pulmonary artery. In other words, the child has two closed circulatory systems, one containing oxygenated blood and one containing oxygen-depleted blood—and the cells of the brain and all the other organs of the body are oxygen starved. The only thing keeping David Morrell alive at this moment is that he has another heart defect, called a VSD, or ventricular septal defect, a hole in the wall between the right and left ventricles. This hole, which Parnell will close during the operation, allows enough mixing of blood between the two chambers to provide a minimal level of oxygen to the cells of the body.

While death is rare enough in the Main O.R. to be a topic of conversation each time it occurs—and it will occur five times this year—this is the kind of operation that could well end unhappily. Aware of that, Peter Walker has made a point of talking to Bridget Lindstrom and the nurses individually before surgery to warn them that this story might not have a happy ending. As Main O.R. head nurse Diana Potenza has observed, although everyone who works in the sixteen rooms is acutely aware that death is always just a crash in blood pressure away, a blood clot, an air bubble, an electrical misfire, an anesthesia reaction or a scalpel slip away, its occurrence is always a shock.

"When somebody dies in the O.R., everybody knows about it," she says. "Word spreads like wildfire. We see it more in the trauma patients, the very sick open heart patients and the vascular patients, like the aneurysm that ruptures and the patient just exsanguinates. You expect those deaths, but they affect you just the same, because you're working, you're doing your best, the whole team, the surgeon, the anesthesiologist, the perfusionists are there, the nursing team . . . When you have a major trauma, everybody just helps out, lends a hand in there, and you're working really hard to save the patient's life, and then when the patient dies, there's that aura of 'Oh, my God!' It just gets very silent. People usually get upset about it. Then the nurses have to take on the fact that they have to do the postmortem care of the patient, clean the patient up while the surgeon notifies the family, and then they have to tell us whether they want to see the patient, because a lot of times the family wants to see the patient before the patient goes downstairs to the morgue. Then my nurses have to deal with seeing the family members and someone has to stay with the family members while they view the body in the recovery room area or in our holding room area. Then we have to inform the morgue to bring the morgue stretcher up, and then the morgue technician takes the body down."

Death in the O.R. is probably harder on new nurses than on anyone else, Potenza says. "I've been in the profession so long, that when somebody dies, I've gone into rooms and let some of the nurses leave because they're so upset dealing with death. I think it's something you never get used to, you just learn how to deal with the situation. I think it's a little easier for O.R. nurses because you're not emotionally involved with the patient and the family. It's easier for them to get over it than the nurses on the floor who get to know the patient over a period of time and get to know the family. We only get to know the patient for about fifteen minutes. But the babies"—she pauses for a moment—"the babies are never easy."

16

10:55 A.M. "This is like putting together a jigsaw puzzle or playing a chess game," plastic surgeon Pam Gallagher is telling the resident working with her in Room 5 to reconstruct Rashid Livingston's mouth and nose. "You're not only thinking about what you do that second, you're thinking about how it's going to affect the next three moves—and that's the hardest thing to teach you. I'm not sure you can teach it, you know what I mean? You can talk about it, but if the person you're teaching doesn't grasp the necessity of planning ahead from a three-dimensional point of view, there isn't much you can do. We've had people like that. ENT [ear, nose, and throat] has some of the same problems when they do reconstructive things. I think spatial relationships are very important, to be able to see things from three dimensions and from different sides. Not to get caught up in left and right. You should be able to look at something from the right, and from the left, and not get upset if they're mirror images of one another."

"But what do you do if it dawns on you all of a sudden that you made a bad move three moves ago? Does that ever happen to you?" asks Roger Pitfick, who less than thirty days ago began his apprenticeship in the Main O.R. as a first-year surgical resident.

"Sure, it happens to me," Gallagher tells him, briefly glancing up over the top of her gold-framed glasses. "What do I do when it happens? Simple, take it all apart and start again. You have to be really impervious, arrogant, to people around you, because they'll say, 'It looks okay.' They want to get the case over. If the nurses are saying there's another case that was supposed to come in an hour ago, you just have to say, 'Tough crap, it doesn't look right to me,' take it apart and do it over again. You've seen this morning, with a lot of this stuff it's 'Well, that stitch wasn't quite good enough.' It's technically all right, but take it out and do it over again. This is a child's face we're talking about, not a chest closure."

Like a methodically worked jigsaw puzzle, the true shape of Rashid's bowed lips has emerged in the past two hours from the pieces that lay hidden from the untrained eye in the misshapen flesh that was his mouth. Gallagher has closed the gap in his upper lip with sutures so fine it is difficult to see them, even in the glaring light washing over Rashid's brown skin. She has placed the stitches in such a way that there is a slight depression, as there should be, defining the midline of the face from upper lip to the base of the nasal septum.

"How do parents deal with this defect?" Pitfick asks her.

"If the fathers get involved, they get very protective, very loving and very hard to deal with"—she laughs—"and very demanding. If they don't get involved, they become rejecting, and it may be years before they get involved. But a lot of that goes away if the family doesn't end up getting divorced. But I don't know if the cleft causes the divorce, or it's a rocky marriage anyway. This is a very correctable condition. It's not like retardation. You have a difficult first year, and then it gets better. I have parents now with their second baby, one who doesn't have the anomaly, and they're concerned that the second baby won't be as good as the first!"

"Are the parents' expectations usually met?"

"I would say ninety percent of the parents are very, very happy," she told him. "Although sometimes they'll say, 'I really like the way it looks, but this isn't quite right.' It's not going to be one hundred percent perfect, I don't care who you are: it's going to be a scar that's a little thick, a nose that's a little crooked. I want them to be able to say that to me and I can say 'Yeah, you're right. We have to see how he grows and what happens. I show them pictures and I show them good results and I show them so-so results. If you can make somebody understand . . . that's why I spend two or three hours with them. But they're always very relieved and very happy because the kids always look a million times better."

As she works on the nose, she explains to the residents: "There's a lot of argument whether you touch a baby's nose at all. Some people worry that you'll have growth distortion. It's part of the argument over whether to go for long-term versus short-term result. I'm going for both long-term and short-term results here. If I really couldn't do this without destroying something, I'd back off and wait. But there are thousands of cases now, fifteen and twenty years out, that show it's better to go ahead than have years of distortion." She slides a minute scalpel blade between the layers of the bridge of the nose, and uses the dull edges of surgical scissors to open the slit she has created. "There are planes you can take advantage of here," she tells the residents, as she separates the layers and uses stitches to bring the nasal cartilage into place. She brings the median of the nose and wings into better position. "You can't expect one stitch to get it all," she says, "because when you correct one deformity, you create another."

Now, at 11:25 A.M., after pulling the right side of the nose more toward the center by placing a single stitch in it, she steps back from the table to survey her work from a distance. "It's not 'poifect,' but it's better," Pam Gallagher says, returning to the table to improve on a job that the toddler's parents, who will never forget what their child looked like when he left his hospital room this morning, would undoubtedly call perfect.

17

When adults would ask four-year-old Pamela Carrasco what she wanted to be when she grew up, they would laugh indulgently when she would tell them she wanted to be a doctor.

"I flirted briefly with wanting to be an archeologist during my nine-to-eleven-year-old phase, but I remember quite distinctly, as early as four, having people laugh when I said I wanted to be a doctor," says Pamela Gallagher, the forty-three-year-old plastic surgeon the little girl became. She laughs as she says that perhaps someone whispered in her ear as she slept, "Be a doctor! Be a doctor!" Something was certainly going on in that comfortable home in East Meadow, on Long Island, given that Gallagher and both her brothers, one older and one younger, went into medicine.

One of fewer than three hundred board-certified female surgeons in the country, Gallagher says she was initially more intrigued by science fiction than factual science. "I didn't do much except read," she says. "I took science to get to medical school. I had a very one-track mind, and whatever I needed to do I did," she says, sitting on the couch in her comfortably furnished, modern office in Garden City. Gallagher recalls that, as a girl interested in science, the only person who tried to block her ambition was a junior high school science teacher who tried to prevent her continuing on in science. "I didn't have a stellar junior high school existence, maybe that's why, but he was very vicious and very adamant about it," she recalls. "I never really understood his opposition, I just attacked it. He was really nasty to me and adamant to the guidance counselor. My father was going to go down and talk to them, but I told him I'd do it. I went in and freaked out. I must have screamed and yelled, because I got exactly what I wanted. My parents' attitude was 'You can do anything you want. So there it is, do it.' " Gallagher says that the first time it occurred to her that there was discrimination against women was the day her father wouldn't let her go with her brother to the Playboy Club in Manhattan. "All of a sudden it hit me like a ton of bricks, that there were differences between girls and boys, and they really couldn't do the same things and get away with it." But Pam Gallagher was raised in what she describes as an "atmosphere of shared jobs, shared responsibilities, shared goals, things like that. My parents sheltered us from other kinds of attitudes." Her father was an engineer and inventor; her mother, a college graduate, was at various times a *Vogue* illustrator, a sculptor and painter, a homemaker and, finally, a medical secretary. So the message, as she says, was "Do what you want to do."

Gallagher believes she chose medicine, rather than some other area of science, because she is a self-described "earth mother type," although she hardly looks it, with her neat, short hairstyle and the crisp, white surgeon's coat she is wearing over a floral dress. "If there was a problem, people brought it to me. It seemed like it was natural to take charge and fix it. I remember as young as three being the leader of the pack on the block. If my friends had trouble, they'd come to me. I see the same thing with both my teenage daughters."

After her high school graduation, Pam Carrasco lived at home and attended nearby Hofstra College, where she minored in art and took psychology courses but, as a premed, worked with the understanding that she had to get straight As. She was vice president of the premed society and shortly after graduation married the president, John Gallagher. "John and I were too stupid to know that you couldn't go to medical school as a couple, so we did it," she says. The couple were accepted everywhere they applied as a couple, and as individuals, including the University of Virginia, the University of Chicago, and Johns Hopkins University. While Hopkins was, and is, one of the top five medical schools in the country, the couple chose Chicago, because they liked the city.

Gallagher says she didn't experience any special difficulties being a woman in medical school in the early 1970s. "I had a friend who was thrown out of Columbia. We suspect it was partially her, but partially the fact that they had too many women in the class that year. But the University of Chicago bent over backward for its female medical students. They were good to us." Which made her intolerant of some of the more strident feminism at the school. She recalls that a number of the women said they weren't planning to repay their loans because they didn't like the treatment women received at Chicago. But Gallagher says she didn't think that was right. "The school went out of its way to make sure its medical students got through. If you failed a course, they gave you the opportunity to make it up. The only thing was that there was a quota system for women, which is what I think annoyed everybody. Twenty percent of the class were women, and this was consistent since 1905—they had five people in the class in 1905 and one was a woman. It was funny. You could look at the pictures of the classes, and it was always twenty percent. There were twenty students on the honor roll and eighteen were women." One of them was Pam

Gallagher. Her husband wasn't one of the twenty, she says, adding, with a laugh, that she believes he was kept off "by affirmative action."

Oddly enough, she believes that rather than making it more difficult to get through medical school, being married made things much easier. "There was a natural bit of loneliness for the people who weren't married or engaged, because they didn't have time to look around too much, they were running ragged all over the place. So a lot of our friends who were single were unhappy about that. And the ones who weren't married to another professional of some sort had marital problems, because the commitment demanded of medical school was all day and all night. There were a lot of divorces in our class the second, third, and fourth year. Then there were also a lot of marriages in our class: I think at least three or four couples found each other in class and married."

When it came time to apply for their residencies, Gallagher says she and her husband "were a little more sophisticated" than they'd been four years earlier. "We really didn't think we'd get the same place, especially with both of us going into surgery," she says. "I'd been committed to psychiatry since high school, that's what I'd wanted to do." But having spent a great deal of time in the University of Chicago's highly respected psychiatry program, she had come to the conclusion that the specialty involved far too much subjective judgment and far too little objective science for her taste. "Another thing was that so much of what they were doing seemed hopeless," she says. "A lot of their patients were hopeless, poor people, like a poor black woman with nine kids, nine different husbands, no education, severe poverty, her last three kids are drug addicts and she's depressed. No kidding. What are you going to do about it? It seemed there was no answer for these patients. You'd meet some of these psychotic patients and you could pour yourself into them forever and never help them. It became very apparent to me that it would tear me apart to try to help them, because there wouldn't be enough of you to go around. It was very sad."

But surgery was a different matter. Like most surgeons, Gallagher chose to go to the O.R. because of the immediate gratification offered there. "In surgery you see a problem, there's frequently a very clear answer, and it ends. You've done something with a concrete, finished product at the end that you can directly affect to a greater or lesser degree. And plastic surgery is a combination of psychiatry, art, and surgery. The poor, depressed fourteen-year-old girl with an ugly nose whose friends make fun of her—rather than give her therapy for two years for her self-esteem, fix the nose and it's over. She feels good, her hair changes, she wears some makeup, her friends say how cute she is and she feels great. It may not be the total answer, but it's part of the answer to what she needs. The children with the cleft lips? If the defect's been corrected by the time people see them and they understand who they are, it never develops into a psychological problem. They don't have any more problems than anybody else has."

Pam Gallagher considered general surgery as a specialty, she recalls, but she "had already pretty much decided I wanted to do plastic surgery." The variety appealed to her. "It was burns, it was reconstructions, it was all kinds of things," she says. "You could take it in any direction you wanted to and keep opening up. A lot of times in surgery you specialize and you're limiting your options. In plastics, you can keep expanding, going where you want to with it."

Getting residencies together turned out to be easier than the couple expected. Normally, fourth-year medical students apply for the residencies they want and then wait at the mercy of the national computerized match program, which takes all the applicants, all the available openings, and matches the choices of the medical students with the choices of the hospitals with residency programs. But the

Gallaghers were able to approach the process differently. "If you were a married couple, you could go outside the matching program," Pam Gallagher explains. "We had done very well in surgery. We were well liked by the chief of surgery at the University of Chicago. So he had a friend at New York Hospital. He called him up and said, 'I have two for you, you want them,' and he said, 'Sure.' But we did go around and look at other programs anyway. The summer between our third and fourth years of medical school, we took a tent, a 1975 Chevy, and $500 and made a huge circle around the United States, camping in national forests and going to our interviews. We'd have all these grubby clothes on and we'd put up the tent, go into the tent and wash up and come out in a suit and a dress, and it was always the same suit and the same dress. People at the campsites would look at us and think, 'Where are they going?' " Gallagher laughs her open, infectious laugh.

Ultimately, the couple stuck with their initial decision to go to New York Hospital, principally because "it was attending taught, not resident-taught"—residents were taught by fully trained surgeons, "so you weren't picking up somebody else's mistake, or misinterpretation, you were getting it directly from the attendings, who were mostly full-time." Gallagher said that, as a woman, she was becoming particularly nervous about placing her future entirely in the hands of other residents, all of whom were male.

The third woman to go through New York Hospital's general surgery residency, and only the second in the plastic surgery program, she says the men didn't "give me too much trouble to my face, but there was a woman two years behind me whom they stomped on, they finally pushed her out." She recalls: "There was a lot of backbiting, a lot of vicious gossip. You'd go to parties to protect yourself. It reminded me of that book, *Lord of the Flies*, with the stressed-out children with no adults to guide them. I remember there was one black resident who a lot of people

were picking on for a while, for no good reason. They
finally realized what they were doing and stopped. But this
one woman, they really bashed her apart. She was very
Southern, very ladylike, real high-class. She didn't wear the
same stupid white uniforms that the rest of us wore—she'd
wear nice white skirts, nice white blouses, she walked with
a little swish. She was at least adequate, if not good. She
was fine. I made the mistake of telling her what was going
on. When she found out, instead of taking it as a warning
to guard her back, she was devastated. It teaches you a
lesson: if people don't know what's going on, don't tell them
about it. Because later on I found out that they were doing
the same thing to me. But by that time I was a third-year
resident and it didn't really matter. I was a senior person.
But I remember being very angry for a whole year. I was
really witchy that year, but then I decided it wasn't worth
it. It only took one or two people to do something like that,
and then it would spread."

Junior residents and interns would be told that " 'She
does this,' or 'She does that,' or 'She's a witch,' or 'She's a
bitch,' " Gallagher says, matter-of-factly. "And then I'd
have interns who were afraid to work with me as a senior
resident because they'd been told I was a bitch. Then they
tried to attack my competence. Rather than say, 'Why didn't
you do this?' they'd just assume I'd screwed up. There was
one incident I particularly recall. We used to live across
the street from the hospital, and I went home for lunch
because there was nothing going on. The interns are supposed to come back, but they'd let us stay at home and take
call. Well, this nurse called to say there was an admission
coming up from Emergency, and I said I'd be over in
fifteen minutes. In reality it was a GI"—gastrointestinal—
"bleeder coming up. She didn't tell me, 'There's a GI
bleeder, get your butt over here.' She was bad to everybody.

"The following year," Gallagher adds, parenthetically,
"another resident punched her out! It was in the middle
of an arrest, and she was sassing him and not responding.

He got so frustrated he decked her. He got thrown out of the hospital for that.

"Anyway, she calls my senior resident and says, 'I told Gallagher to come. But she said she'd be there in twenty minutes.' That guy hated my guts for two years, rather than call me on the carpet then and there. Two years later we had a fight and I found out what happened.

"But I have a layer of rubber around me that's very thick. It took three years for them to break through and get me really crazy. What got to me wasn't the nitpicking behind my back, it was that they had frightened the interns so badly about me that nobody wanted to work with me. That's what got me crazy. My feeling was always that you worked as hard as you could, if you did a good job there was nothing anybody could say. If you were a good girl, Daddy was going to pat you on the head. It took me three years to realize that that's not how it worked. It strengthened me a lot. But it broke some people. There's also a lot of divide-and-conquer. For instance, there's this thing called the 'queen bee syndrome.' A lot of the women felt that if they got through, and they survived, they shouldn't reach back and help the women behind them. As a matter of fact, they're going to step on the one behind them. That way they'll be the only woman, and be the queen bee, not realizing that that was a way to isolate them, not support them. There were a couple of women who came through behind me who played that game, and didn't realize how isolated they were, how damaged they were, and how despised they were—including by the guys who were hanging all around them. It was very sad to see that isolating process. They thought they'd be one of the boys. And they were made to think they were one of the boys, but I had a 'boy' who told me what they were, and it wasn't one of the boys. I think having a husband who was in the whole process, and could clarify it from the other side, was a big help."

Gallagher says she learned at a very young age to deal

with sexual harassment because everything she did "was around boys. I did karate and judo as my sports in high school," she says. "In med school I was surrounded by boys. So you register it at a very subliminal level, but you learn not to react to it. There are very subtle signals you give back, saying you're interested or not interested. Well, I learned very young, as my daughter has, not to react to other people's signals. So you could exist in that world without being bothered too much, except by people who didn't want to read your answer.

"So I only had one real groping incident," she says, able to laugh about it now. "I was pregnant in October of my intern year. It wasn't totally unplanned. Our feeling was you had to start some time, so you might as well let the chips fall where they may. We were already married seven years. When we looked ahead, there was no good time. We had two salaries, we had a nice little apartment, we could afford a housekeeper. It was sort of like, if it happened, it happened. We were making like $9,000 each. But we only had to pay the housekeeper $150 a week. So my salary paid for the housekeeper and the rent, and his paid for everything else. Anyway, I had my baby in August. She was due July 31, she came August 13, and I was back to work September 1 in the Emergency Room, twenty-four hours on, twelve hours off. Breasts out to here, milk coming in, pain like you wouldn't believe, and I'd never heard of getting wrapped—they didn't teach you that in medical school, but the nurses in the E.R. taught me about wrapping my breasts. But if you asked people if I was out on maternity leave, they'd say yes, not because I was, but because that was what they'd expected to see."

As perverse as it may seem, the one sexual harassment incident occurred when she was seven months pregnant. "I was on the thoracic service and the guy who was the chief resident was from Jordan and he hated my guts. He hated women period, except in their proper place, which was whatever he decided it was at the time. But he hated me especially. I had this irritating cough, because I had asthma during pregnancy. It used to make him crazy. We used to have to sleep like a bunch of gerbils in the I.C.U., and I'd be coughing. Well, during surgery, I'd have to hold all the hooks and things, and he would rub up against my stomach. It was really gross. I never told my husband, because he would have decked him." Gallagher says the man involved tried to cause her trouble over the quality of her work, or paperwork, but friends would always back her up. "A lot of my fellow interns were like that, friends, who didn't treat women and men differently," she says. "The other people were dinosaurs, and we couldn't understand their attitudes. It was the next generation coming through that was supportive, the young guys were much more supportive than the older guys were. And I was in competition with the younger guys, because there were only like six chief resident's positions and there were twelve or fifteen interns."

Because she had managed to do an extraordinary amount of general surgery in her first three years, Pam Gallagher was able to move from general surgery into a plastic surgery residency after three years, rather than the usual five. After completing the two years of subspecialty training in June 1979, she joined Long Island Plastic Surgery Associates, in Garden City, one of the nation's largest plastic surgery groups, and began reverse commuting to her home in Manhattan while her husband, in training as a vascular surgeon, completed his training. The couple then moved to Long Island, and John Gallagher, who was doing a fellowship in vascular surgery in New Jersey, came home every other weekend. And in the midst of all that, Pam Gallagher took six weeks off to have her now-seven-year-old son. "They used to call him the $40,000 baby," she says, because of the income lost to the group during those six weeks of maternity leave.

Gallagher says she joined the group because of the backup it afforded her. In her first years she could have a partner present for many of her procedures, her way of acknowledging that there's still a learning curve after formal training ends.

"It wasn't that I wasn't an experienced surgeon, because I was. But when I spent my first five years in private practice, it scares you so much that the night before you go to the books and you look everything up and you re-read it again and you look to see if there's anything new," she says. "The pressure's there, the fear that you're going to hurt the patient, that you're going to do anything that's irrevocable. To this day I still prepare the night before. When you're doing cosmetic surgery, what makes it scary is that you're taking someone who's normal and you're trying to make them better normal. In my mind, for myself, there's no excuse for a complication, there's no excuse for a little scar, there's no excuse for a cut nerve, a paralysis, a severe infection, a hematoma that causes that loss of skin, a disfiguring finish. Because you're just taking something that's all right and trying to make it better, so you'd better, so you darn well better try the hardest you can to do that. That's why I'm very slow to pick up a new 'fad' that comes through, because I want to make sure that there's five years of experience and everybody else has had the bad experiences that I'm not going to have. I guess the world has to have some arrogant people who don't give a shit—excuse the expression—and then the rest of us. And most of the surgeons I know feel the way I do. The other thing is that you do get a sense of confidence. For instance, if I approach a nose now, I've done so many noses that . . . I can dream noses in my head. It gets to a point where it's never routine, but it's comfortable. I remember with breast reductions when I started in practice. I wasn't comfortable. It didn't feel right handling the tissue, I'd seen too many complications as a resident. I was scared. Now breast reductions are something that I'm comfortable with. I'm very surprised if I have a complication. Breast reductions are very common. And I get a lot of young girls who are very asymmetrical, like one's a C and one's nothing. I get one every two weeks, or three weeks. They come in the spring, bathing suit weather. Obviously I'm going to get more than somebody else is, because a lot of them are young girls, thirteen, or fourteen, and they're not going to go to a male doctor. They don't want their mother to see them, so they'd die if a guy saw them."

Although she says she gets the greatest satisfaction from the kind of reconstructive work she does for children like Rashid Livingston—from whose parents she will accept what little Medicaid will pay of the normal $5,500 fee— she claims to enjoy all of plastic surgery. "Face-lifts are irritating, because they're long and they're scary in some places. But everybody can relate to the desire to have one. Who wants to look ugly? Why is there something wrong or immoral about not looking ugly? I consider myself a very involved person religiously and ethically and morally. But I don't see what's wrong with helping somebody feel better about themselves, whether they're old and ugly or young and ugly. You can sit down and say, 'It's wrong for society to judge somebody by what they look like from the outside.' Well, it's all well and good to say it, but the point is they do. You comb your hair, you take a bath, you put a ribbon in your hair. That's part of being human, too. I have one lady who really brings it home to me. She's a secretary and she used to be a hairdresser. She had kind of a hard marriage, and when her husband died she saved up her pennies for her face-lift, and her eyebrow lift and her eyelids and her dermabrasion, a whole rejuvenation process. It took her two years to get everything done she wanted, because it was expensive and she had to save her money. She told me she never wanted to look old. I've been taking care of her for about eleven years—a little tuck here, a little lift there. She said, 'When people are old, nobody respects you.' Now she's about seventy-two and she looks about fifty. When she goes to the hospital—she's had breast cancer and she's had to have radiation and this, that, and the other thing—people don't call her a 'little old lady.' They call the woman in the bed next to her who's ten years younger a 'little old lady.' And they talk over that person's head, and they talk around her. But when they address my patient, they talk to her face, and they look at her and they listen to her views because she looks like a fifty-year-old woman, not a seventy-year-old."

Gallagher is quick to acknowledge that part of her motivation for going into medicine was the freedom it gives her. "I wanted to be my own boss. While that's never really true, I think you do have more independence and control of your life than an employee in business. You can't get fired. I'm responsible for myself. I can set my office hours. I usually end up working more than I want because if I have a consult, then I wind up with more hours tomorrow. I never wanted a routine, nine to five, what I considered boring job. And a lot of the changes are turning medicine into that. What's going to happen is it's going to change the attitude. One thing about capitalism is if you put the hours in, you get paid for it."

Balancing a full-time medical career with motherhood is difficult, Pam Gallagher says, laughing once again and noting that "you're taking time away from me with my kids right now. Some times are worse than others. This summer has been very bad. So I've told my office I'm taking off two afternoons a week. If my patients have to wait three months, they have to wait. If they won't wait, I can't worry about that. I get coerced a lot, like I'm going to take off this day to be with my kids and then I get pushed because I'm told that a patient needs to see me, so I figure I can drop in in the morning and take the afternoon off, and I used to give in to that. I'm getting better at not giving in to that. But I did it a lot this summer, and my kids were pointing it out to me, so I've decided I won't do it. My oldest daughter was the child of my internship, so she had the least time with me initially, but she also had the best housekeeper we ever had. It's sort of an experiment. Nobody really knows what's going to happen with the stresses of working mothers. Maybe this generation of kids will be screwballs when they grow up. We talk about 'father hunger,' maybe there'll be 'mother hunger,' too. But my kids seem to be fine. My daughter's talked sometimes about being angry about it. But she used to get angry when people would say, 'Your father's a doctor?' And she'd say, 'My mother's a doctor, too.' "

18

11:35 A.M. It had been a tight squeeze, thirty minutes ago, when third-year resident Matthew Prince held open the door to O.R. 1 for the bed bearing seventeen-year-old Andre Fogarassi. Room 1 is one of the nine, smaller, sixteen-by-twenty-foot operating spaces, and with the operating table in the center of the room, the anesthesia equipment and instrument stands, and the transport bed with the seven people surrounding it, there was little space left to maneuver. The trip from one of the patient floors to the Main O.R. might normally require only a transporter to push the gurney. But in this case, because Andre is comatose, needs artificial support to breathe, and is being moved on a bed, the trip to the O.R. required the additional help of anesthesiologist Leo Penzi and two nurses, who were joined by vascular surgeon Larry Scher and a resident.

"What happened to him?" asked scrub nurse Anne Bullard, as she helped slide Andre's limp body from the bed to the O.R. table.

"He was in the backseat of a car," Penzi told her.

"Did he go through the windshield?"

"The back window," said Penzi, who was using an Ambu

Bag to breathe by hand for Andre, squeezing on the black, football-shaped bag attached to his tracheostomy fitting, forcing oxygen into the youngster's lungs.

"The back window?! Oh my God!"

The sheets covering Andre's body were removed, and it was then possible to see why he had been brought to Room 1 this morning: his left leg is dead, rotting, from about six inches below the knee to the bottom of his foot. From knee to sole, this limb that powered Andre Fogarassi's bicycle, that carried him downstairs to breakfast every morning and along school corridors, that kicked a soccer ball and stole bases ranges in color from normal beige to green-tinged reddish brown to black. An incision made three days ago in a vain attempt to save the leg is still open, and the tibia is partially visible.

While the nurses finished cleaning the area above the knee, and wrapped the dead foot and ankle in the clear plastic that would eventually hold the amputated limb, Scher went to the scrub sink. "I want to talk to Dr. Harvey before I begin," he told the two residents scrubbing with him. "It's a philosophical thing: If there's any chance he'll ever be able to use it again, we'd like to save the knee, do something good for his parents. But his chances are . . ." He paused, shaking his head. "So maybe we should just take it above the knee, not take the chance we have to bring him in again."

But unable to reach his colleague Scher went with his gut feeling that he should make the attempt to save Andre Fogarassi's knee, and now, at 11:35, he makes his initial incision, about four inches below the knee and two inches above the gangrenous area. He works carefully, preserving enough skin and healthy tissue to produce a usable stump, which will be helpful in the unlikely event the youngster ever regains consciousness, and then function, to the point where he can once again walk. Thirteen minutes after

Scher and Matthew Prince begin cutting, Penzi increases
the amount of fluid he is giving the patient, attempting to
make up for ever-increasing blood loss.

The amputation of Andre Fogarassi's leg may be taking
place in a modern O.R. in a high-tech medical center, and
the latest therapeutic chemistry may make it pain-free and
allow the surgeons to take the time needed to do the job
right, but the act itself is a trip through time. This is surgery
at its most basic, as it was practiced in tents at Gettysburg,
in the surgeon's cockpit between decks on the *Bonhomie
Richard*, in the mud of Agincourt—even beneath the walls
of Jericho. When surgeons, barbers, or shamen could do
nothing else, they could amputate limbs. All it took was a
sharp blade, strong arms, and a strong stomach. Which is
all it takes this July morning.

"The Gigli please," says Scher, and Anne Bullard hands
him the Gigli saw, a crude but effective device invented by
Leonardo Gigli, a nineteenth-century Italian gynecologist
who needed a good blade to cut through the pubic bone.
The saw consists of a flexible wire imbedded with razor-
sharp teeth, much like the kind of survival saw that can be
ordered from the L.L. Bean catalog. It is held, and pulled
back and forth in even strokes, by two removable steel and
wood handles that look like old-fashioned skate hooks. Matthew Prince slips the wire blade beneath the exposed tibia,
attaches the handles, and saws. It takes him only thirty-
five seconds to sever the bone. Scher then hands medical
student Josh Quittner a bone cutter, which looks like giant
toenail clippers, and tells him to cut through the smaller
fibula. When Quittner fails to cut all the way through, Scher
kids him, saying, "You're a disgrace! You're from Brooklyn,
right? That's what they do in Brooklyn, break people's
bones."

It is 12:05. Scher lifts Andre Fogarassi's leg off the table
and hands it to circulating nurse Ellen Reynolds, who
places it on the specimen table. As the surgical team finishes
the procedure, closing the wound at the new end of Andre

Fogarassi's leg, the discarded portion lies forgotten in the corner of the room, a pathology specimen tag lying next to it. And on the same table lies the youngster's chart, with an initial admitting note, written forty days before:

> Motor vehicle collision. Depressed skull fracture. Subdural and epidural hematoma. Partial fracture. Contusions and abrasions. No fault.

The last two words do not reflect someone's moral or legal judgment; they simply refer to the state's no-fault auto insurance plan, which will pay for Andre Fogarassi's care up to $50,000—an amount long ago exceeded.

"Well," says Scher, as he, Prince, and Quittner finish their work, "at least we have some good news for the parents. We saved the knee."

19

12:06 P.M. Many plastic surgeons would have considered the repair of Rashid Livingston's lip and nose completed thirty minutes ago, but Pam Gallagher wasn't ready to quit. "You have to go for better now," she told the residents. "Otherwise you kick yourself three months from now. When you've made such a big change, the temptation is to let it go."

To the untrained eye, there is nothing left for Gallagher to do: the tattered pieces of flesh that were the top portion of the baby's mouth have been joined together, in a virtually seamless flow, to form a perfectly bowed upper lip, and the broken lines of the nose have been joined together with minute stitches so that the right and left nostrils flair as mirror images of each other. But the daughter of the fashion illustrator turned sculptor is not quite finished.

She snips about an eighth of an inch off a Silastic, translucent, infant urinary catheter and then places the piece of tubing inside the right wing of the nose to keep it from collapsing. "I'm giving you the five-minute warning," she tells her circulating nurse, indicating that it's time to notify the front desk that Room 5 will soon be available for the next scheduled surgeon and procedure.

Gallagher next cuts a second piece of catheter and sews it to the surface of the nose, above the first piece, connecting the two with a stitch. "This," she announces, "is the plastic in plastic surgery. They used to use gold beads, but they damaged the skin. So now we use plastic. Which makes sense."

Now Pam Gallagher looks down at Rashid Livingston and beams, finally satisfied with her work. "Welcome to the world, new baby," she says, softly. "Hopefully, you'll be more welcome now."

20

12:10 P.M. Given Jack Hannan's terror at having an injection in his wrist and having a rubber tube snaked up his nose, it's lucky he can't see himself at this moment, with neurosurgeon Nancy Epstein poised to make her initial incision in the back of his neck.

The upper end of the operating table has been raised to create a kind of chair, and Hannan is asleep in a sitting position. His shoulders, neck, and head extend above the upper edge of the surgical chair, and his head is held upright by being literally screwed, and then taped, into an erector set-like frame that rises from the side of the surgical table about midway down and, using a series of metal rods and fittings, extends toward Hannan. The front half of his head is cradled in a padded, metal, C-shaped brace, held in position by two set-screws, one on the right and one on the left, with yards of tape wrapped around the brace and Hannan's head.

Twin, white, translucent tubes snake from the fitting on the end of his endotracheal tube to the $50,000 Narkomed 2A anesthesia machine at the top left side of the table—viewed from the head. A mass of multicolored wire spaghetti, leading to an additional $55,000 in monitoring equipment, winds its way across Hannan's body and spills over the side of the O.R. table. All of this equipment allows anesthesiologist Fred Fabiano to keep Hannan breathing, asleep, pain-free, amnesic, fully oxygenated, in fluid balance, with his blood pressure and heart rate within proper parameters. Fabiano is also using a sonarlike cardiac doppler to monitor the sound of blood flowing through Hannan's heart. There is an increased possibility, when the patient is in this sitting position, that a potentially fatal air bubble may make its way into the heart, thus the use of the Doppler, which will alert Fabiano to any changes in the sound of blood flowing through that natural pump.

All other preparations completed, the anesthesiologist takes a flashlight and ducks beneath the mountain of blue paper and green cloth drapes covering Hannan's body and tapes the patient's eyes shut.

"Ready to go?" asks Nancy Epstein. She then takes an electric cautery and makes a four-inch vertical incision just to the right of the midline of Hannan's neck, above the two cervical vertebrae known as C-6 and C-7.

A decade ago, when she joined her father's neurosurgical practice, Nancy Epstein was, not surprisingly, known far and wide as "Joe Epstein's daughter," which was admittedly an improvement on the name Olive Oyl, which was hung on the thin, intense, 5′11″ woman, who wears her black hair in a bun, during her neurosurgery residency at New York University Medical Center in Manhattan. But today, the twelfth of twenty-eight women ever to be board-certified in neurosurgery, with teaching appointments at both Cornell University Medical School and Columbia University, chapters contributed to fourteen books and her name on almost fifty scientific papers, Nancy Epstein is no longer known as her seventy-four-year-old father's daughter. The day has long since passed when an attending neurosurgeon at Long Island Jewish Hospital, where Nancy Epstein also practices, would even think of doing something so gauche as to pull the reflex hammer from the pocket of Epstein's white coat and ask her if her Daddy gave it to her to play with. (Epstein recalls she simply looked down at her rude colleague, "who was about five-two," and curtly noted that his action and remark "were entirely inappropriate.") In fact, Nancy Epstein is now so established in neurosurgery circles that the tables have truly turned, with the widely respected Joseph Epstein sometimes being referred to as "Nancy Epstein's father."

As a child, Epstein used to join her father when he made rounds at the hospitals at which she now practices. She recalls them as much smaller institutions, where she used to sometimes play on the lawns. "Every Thursday night we'd go out for Chinese dinner and I would get to go into the recovery room, because after dinner my father would check on the patients he had operated on. Then, Saturday mornings, as I got older, I got to go on rounds with him, and he took me into the O.R. when I was about fifteen. There was probably an older age limit, but I was so tall—I was five-eleven by the time I was eleven—so it didn't really make much difference in terms of people questioning my age."

When Joe Epstein went to visit his daughter for Harvest Festival, the fall of her junior year at Putney, the ultra-liberal prep school in Vermont that she attended for two years, she announced to him that it made no sense for her to spend an additional year in high school. She was ready instead to begin the long march to her career in neurosurgery. She argued that she had already taken most of the courses Putney had to offer. Four years of college, four years of medical school and six or seven years of residency lay ahead of her. So the following September, after a summer spent working as a volunteer teacher in South America—and after meeting a Peace Corps volunteer who would shortly become her first husband—she was off to college at Barnard a year early.

There were about thirty women out of one hundred and

twenty students in Epstein's medical school class at Columbia University's College of Physicians and Surgeons, and
their degree of acceptance depended upon the subspecialty
they planned to pursue, Epstein says. "Women were already integrated—and I don't think it's changed very
much—into pediatrics, and ob-gyn. As long as it wasn't
'important,' it was okay for the women to go into it. I taught
a course for undergraduates at Columbia this fall with my
husband [her second husband, who she met after her brief,
first marriage, is a professor of psychology and former
Columbia dean], on physiological modes of electrical monitoring. We had five students and one was a woman premed." Epstein asked the young woman what she was interested in, and when the student replied, "Medicine," Epstein asked which specialty. "She said 'I want to be a
dermatologist.' I said, 'Why bother going to college?' " re-
counts Epstein, who has the typical surgeon's disdain of
some of the medical subspecialties into which women are
often channeled. But she worked on the student, and "now
she wants to come into the O.R. If I could save one mind,
it's worth it." Epstein laughs at her own hyperbole.

"But I'll never forget, when I was applying to medical
schools I went to one institution and they asked, 'How is
the fact that you're a woman going to prevent you from
pursuing a successful medical career?' I said, 'Well, I guess
the interview's over.' And at two places they asked what
kind of birth control I used. I remember, one of them asked
'What kind of birth control do you use?' " and Epstein,
without missing a beat, shot back, "Rhythm." "They knew
I was married, so they said, 'What are you going to do
about children?' 'Nothing,' I said, and they drew a blank.
'Who ever said I was interested in having children?' " she
said to them. "Having children is not something I've ever
thought about," she says, noting that she and her second
husband, to whom she has been married for more than
fifteen years, have their days and nights filled without children. For Nancy Epstein, life is work, and work is life. "The

students are my children," she says, "and that's as close as I want to get."

Jack Hannan's operation is moving almost unbelievably quickly, without incident. Twenty-two minutes after making her first incision, Epstein announces that she's reached the spinal cord and begins removing the exposed fragments of Hannan's two herniated disks, the pads that separate and cushion the vertebrae. For all the young accountant's fears, the operation itself, which can take as long as four hours, will take less than an hour and a half, in part because of all the time spent in preparation and, in part, because his injury couldn't be more straightforward.

21

12:35 P.M. "Hey, Peter, did I tell you I ran into Ralph at the cardiac meeting?" asks Vinnie Parnell, without looking up from Baby Morrell's heart.

"No kidding? Where is he now, Des Moines or someplace like that?"

"Lincoln, Nebraska, believe it or not. Joined a group out there and, with his good luck, one of the two partners left six months later. Two weeks after that the senior partner died, so now Ralph's the senior partner."

"He always had great luck. Is he still an SOB?" Peter Walker asks.

"That'll never change either. I remember we were at a resident's evaluation meeting, I think his fourth year, and his name came up. As we went around the table, one guy after another got up to give his comments, and one would say about Ralph, 'He's really arrogant,' another would say, 'He's too cold,' another would say, 'He's incredibly conceited.' Then another said, 'He's technically very good, but he's too arrogant.' Then three or four of the general surgeons each said, 'He'll never make it, he's not right for surgery.' Then they came to one of the cardiac guys, who'd been taking all this in, and he jumped up and said, 'Perfect!

He'll make a great cardiac surgeon!' " There is loud laughter from all corners of Room 3, relieving the natural tension of surgery.

The Morrell baby has been "on the pump" for one hour and twelve minutes, which means that for that period of time the infant has, in effect, been dead: his blood is being oxygenated, filtered, and circulated by two of three Stockert-Shiley mechanical pumps that do the most vital work of the heart-lung machine that perfusionist Bridget Lindstrom is manning. A clear, flexible, Silastic canula, or hose, runs from the femoral artery in the infant's thigh, to one of the pumps, where a roller squeezes and releases the hose at a fixed rate, drawing blood through it. After being cleansed by one of the disposable filters Lindstrom attached prior to surgery, and then being oxygenated, the blood is pumped back to the baby through a second canula stitched into the aorta above the area where Vinnie Parnell will be working. The heart-lung machine is also used to regulate the temperature of the blood, heating and chilling it, and also includes a device called a cell saver, which collects and filters and stores the blood that is bleeding into the chest cavity as Parnell operates, reducing the amount of blood substitutes and donated blood the infant will need. Additionally, the heart-lung machine is used to pump an ice-cold fluid, called cardioplegia, to the body, chilling the heart, to keep it from beating during surgery and to protect the cells from damage.

At 11:23 Parnell gave the word to Bridget Lindstrom. "Bridget, you ready?"

"Ready."

"Okay, let's go."

Lindstrom reached up from her seat and removed scissorlike surgical clamps from the lines leading to and from the infant's body, and bright red blood flowed through the lines. At the same time, Walker turned off the ventilator portion of the anesthesia machine, as the pump was oxygenating the blood and the infant no longer needed the mechanical respirator. "We're at half flow," Lindstrom told the surgeon.

"Okay, stay there," Parnell said, checking the purse string sutures holding the line in place in the aorta. "Take the blood temp down."

"To twenty?"

"Sixteen would be good," replies the surgeon, telling the perfusionist to chill the blood to 16 degrees centigrade, or about 61 degrees Fahrenheit.

"Do you have some cardioplegia ready for us?" surgeon's assistant Dom DiCapua asked Lindstrom at 11:35. "Okay, start your cardioplegia now." After placing crushed ice around the heart to stop it entirely, Parnell took a small piece of Gortex fabric and cut out a piece about the size of a dime. As he placed a hair-size suture in the patch, Peter Walker worked on the anesthesia record, noting all drugs and fluids he had given Baby Morrell to that point.

"Bridget? The blood temperature's still sixteen and the rectal's still twenty?" asked Parnell.

"Yes."

At that moment Rosco "Rocky" Rossi, the anesthesiologist "running the floor"—coordinating all anesthesia services—today, brings Walker a letter to sign that the anesthesia group's administrator didn't want to sign for him. "She's signed for me enough before," Walker said, slightly irritated.

"But this isn't a hotel register, Peter," Parnell gibed.

"Thanks a lot," Walker responded, laughing.

"All right," Parnell announced at 12:09, "we've done all the preliminaries, we'll start the real operation in just a minute." Again, everyone in the room laughed, knowing that, having closed the hole between the infant's ventricles, he has already successfully completed a routine pediatric cardiac procedure.

But now, at 12:35, as he slices through Baby Morrell's aorta, severing it from the heart, his main work does, indeed, lie ahead of him. Parnell cuts down on the stump of the aorta and frees a small portion of the main coronary artery. "You can't kink it, can't twist it, can't compress it. You can't look cross-eyed at this or you've had it," he says. Next he uses a suture to mark the position of the valve inside the pulmonary artery, the valve that will be the aortic valve when the operation is over.

Performing what is known as the LeCompte Maneuver, the surgeon tucks the aorta behind the pulmonary artery, bringing it to the back side of the heart. He then runs a series of minute sutures through the stump of the severed pulmonary artery and the now-free aorta. How many sutures? "I hope I put the right number in," he replies, matter-of-factly, "just enough so it doesn't leak at the end." He completes his connection of the aorta to the stump of the pulmonary artery and announces: "It's good-bye and good luck. Once this is stitched and in place, you can't get to it if it's leaking. People used to say the soul resides in the pineal gland. Nowadays, we say it's below the pulmonary artery and the aorta."

22

12:53 P.M. In the hallway outside Room 2, Leo Schmidt is refusing to be anesthetized. The sixty-seven-year-old retired contractor is scheduled for a skin graft this afternoon to repair an infected area in his arm that was opened up and irrigated. "I don't mind having the tube put in, but I don't want to wake up with it in," he is telling anesthesiologist Andrew Chang.

"You are afraid of waking up with it?" Chang asks.

"I'm scared to death," says Schmidt.

"How are you doing?" plastic surgeon Joseph Feinberg asks, quietly, stepping up behind Chang. "Are you winning it or losing it?"

"Losing it," the anesthesiologist tells him. This is not going well. For the past twenty minutes he has been unsuccessfully attempting to calm Schmidt, who, at this point, would rather have the surgery canceled than risk waking up attached to a mechanical ventilator. Schmidt has reason to be fearful: it took four attempts to insert his endotracheal tube, or intubate him, for an earlier procedure, and he suffered cardiac arrest and almost died during the fourth attempt.

"Mr. Schmidt? Dr. Feinberg," says the surgeon, laying

his hand on the patient's left shoulder. "How are you doing?"

"Not good."

"Look, Mr. Schmidt, we'll get the tube out. There's no promises, you know that, but they'll do their damnedest. Let's let these gentlemen do their job."

"Can't we put this operation off a while?" the white-haired patient pleads.

"No," the surgeon tells him, "that will just make things worse. The reason I want to do this now is the area around the elbow, where it was irrigated, is drying out. Your wife wants you to have this done, Mr. Schmidt. She's out in the waiting area." Without waiting for Schmidt to respond, the surgeon gestures to the transporter to wheel the gurney into Room 2, and Andrew Chang follows behind.

Two doors down the hall, in Room 1A, Michael Setzen has begun the work of rebuilding Lillian Paskow's esophagus. The laryngectomy and radical neck resection procedure, expected to take about seven hours, has moved along so smoothly that it is winding down almost three hours ahead of schedule.

It was exactly an hour ago that Michael Setzen and his partner began removing the larynx itself. "It may look like we're moving briskly," Setzen said then, "and we are. But we're being cautious at the same time. Any one of these vessels can bleed excessively. This procedure can result in weakness of the tongue, lip, shoulder, stroke, a fistula, swallowing problems, or death. That's why I always tell people to go home and think about this, get a second opinion. Hello, Darlene, come to see your fellow smoker?" Setzen switched conversational tracks as nurse Darlene Farber came into the room, a box of Camel filters pushing out the breast pocket of her surgical scrubs. Instead of responding to Setzen, she asked the circulating nurse when Lillian Paskow would be ready for a bed in the Post Anesthesia Care Unit—the Recovery Room.

Setzen ignored being ignored, and continued: "Smoking causes chronic irritation of the larynx, so they get swollen vocal cords, hoarseness—and as they continue to smoke, this larynx is being bathed in the nicotine over twenty years—thirty years . . . and then things develop. Had Mrs. Paskow come to me three weeks after she'd noticed hoarseness, we could have done a simple, sophisticated laser resection of her tiny vocal cord tumor, left the rest of her larynx intact, not had to do the bilateral, radical neck dissections, maybe not had to do radiation therapy, and this lady would have only had that laser laryngoscopy and resection of a small tumor. It could have been an outpatient procedure. When it's late in the disease, we have to do the major resection. But a lot of people that have been smokers have had hoarseness since young adulthood. They continue to be hoarse. They say, 'I'm a smoker, I just have chronic laryngitis.'

"I see a lot of patients and I see a lot of people with simple problems, sinus problems, nasal problems, voice changes," said the thirty-seven-year-old Setzen. "But when I see this kind of patient . . . I've done a fiber-optic examination, I see this cancer in the larynx—because we can diagnose it then and there. I know what the problem is. It looks like a cancer. I then feel her neck and it's this hard mass. And I know it's a metastasis. I've got to sit back and say to myself, 'I've got a problem here. This patient needs major surgery. She's going to be devastated by the surgery initially. She's not going to be able to comprehend what I tell her when I tell her about the procedure and what it's all about, what the potential risks are, what she's going to be like postoperatively. It's a mammoth task for me. So, as I said, what I'll do is I'll have them come back a number of times. When I talk to her the first time I don't tell her it's a cancer, because I can be wrong. I need a pathologic diagnosis. So I tell her, 'I see a tumor in the larynx, I'm very concerned about it. We're going to need to biopsy this.' And the minute you mention 'biopsy,' the question

is 'Do you think it's malignant?' If I think it's malignant, I
say to them, 'I think it may be malignant, but I cannot be
sure,' because I want them to realize this is serious—don't
go away and come back to me in six months. I want you
to go away and come back immediately and let's schedule
this procedure. So they know this is serious. I then spend
a lot of time talking to her and her family about what's
going on in my mind. I personally try not to keep secrets
in these kinds of cases. In other cases, that aren't as significant, we can say less. But I think in this kind of situation,
she's the patient, she's going to be the one to deal with this
kind of procedure, no one else. Not me, not her husband,
and not her family. So I personally would rather tell her
everything. I don't necessarily say how serious the disease
is and that she's gonna die. I give them a lot of hope. I
say, 'We're going to take care of it, and if it is malignant
we'll do this procedure and I anticipate we're going to cure
you. We are going ahead with the understanding we're
going to cure you. We're not just doing this operation with
a hope, we're going to cure you.'

"We're going to bring them through the operation," said
Setzen, who received his medical education in his native
South Africa, and then did a second residency and specialty
training in this country, at the prestigious Cleveland Clinic
and Barnes Hospital, in St. Louis. "The chances of us kill-
ing a patient on the operating table from a major head and
neck operation are extremely remote. I've never had a
patient die on the table and I hope never to. Depending
on the stage of the disease, I think that for her, her chances
of five-year survival are in excess of seventy-five percent."
Setzen said that when he tells patients that, they question
the value of the procedure. The alternative, he points out,
is a 100 percent chance of death in the near term. "Then
I let them go home and talk to their families, get a second
opinion. I think second opinions in a situation like this are
important, because they want to see another doctor un-
related to me. 'What do you think? Do you think this is a

serious problem? Do you think I need to have that kind of operation? What are my chances for cure?' I think they need to hear it from somebody else.

"Well, Jim," he then told the chief resident, changing the subject back to the work at hand, "you've done a terrific dissection here." Earlier, outside Sullivan's hearing, Setzen had noted that surgery can be taught destructively, by tearing the residents down to the bare roots of their being and rebuilding them as surgeons, or it can be taught by praise and positive reinforcement. Setzen, who was himself the object of the former kind of training, believes in the latter, kinder, technique.

With the trachea, and the esophagus immediately behind it, fully exposed, Setzen took scalpel in hand and sliced through the trachea, revealing the off-white endotracheal tube used for anesthesia. The surgeon then pulled the plastic tube out, through Lillian Paskow's mouth, temporarily removing her from the respirator, placed a new tube directly into the lower section of the trachea, and had her reconnected to the machine—all in less than forty-five seconds. He then sliced into Paskow's esophagus, revealing the growth of the tumor in the wall of that passage, and cut free about three inches of trachea—and vocal cords—esophagus and malignant mass.

Now, as he begins the business of reconstructing the esophagus, it is possible to look up Lillian Paskow's eviscerated neck and see light coming down from her open mouth. It is difficult, at this point, to believe that she will ever leave O.R. alive, much less "start liquids by mouth and a soft diet in ten to fourteen days," as Setzen tells Sullivan. To replace the missing section of esophagus, and complete the passage from Paskow's mouth to her stomach, Setzen forms a tube of the layers of muscle along the sides of the esophagus, drawing them together with a Dexon suture, which will dissolve in about six weeks. He uses a single running stitch on each layer of the new esophagus, with about twenty individual stitches making up each closure.

Next, Setzen and Sullivan bring muscle around from the back of Lillian Paskow's neck and attach it in the front of her neck, using it to cover and protect the carotid artery, which they worked so hard to preserve during the operation. "If she got a leak, and got saliva on the carotid, she could have a carotid blow out," says Setzen, explaining that the saliva could erode the thin wall of the artery. "Then, after all this work, she'd be gone."

It is now 1:18 P.M., four hours and fifty-seven minutes after Michael Setzen directed Jim Sullivan to make the first incision in Lillian Paskow's throat. Setzen releases the clamps gripping the sutures that are holding the skin of Paskow's throat and neck and pulls the flap back into place. Then he matches up the marks he made before surgery, on the flap and on the surrounding tissue, and completes the process of reconstructing Lillian Paskow. It will be almost another hour before the drainage tubes are in place, the new tracheostomy fitting is ready—allowing Paskow to breathe, and speak, through a hole in her throat—the bandaging is complete, all the other external work is finished, and Paskow is sent to the Recovery Room. The surgical heavy lifting is completed. But Lillian Paskow's life is still very much at risk.

23

1:20 P.M. Two environmental service workers have just finished removing the detritus created by the day's first "cabbage"—coronary artery bypass graft—from Room 4, the one O.R. dedicated to cardiac surgery. The official line at North Shore is that "there is no unimportant job." It is said that what these workers, who despite their euphemistic job title are at the bottom of the Main O.R.'s rigidly hierarchical staff pyramid, do is, in its way, "just as important as what the surgeon does." The chief of surgery, Tony Tortolani, says that. The head nurse, Diana Potenza, says that. The chief of anesthesia, Peter Walker, says that. North Shore's *eminence grise*, eighty-three-year-old general surgeon John Mountain, says that. With a straight face. Amazingly enough, it's true. The environmental service worker, an employee who is probably male and Hispanic and may have a poor grasp of English, may earn in an hour about three percent of what a cardiac surgeon earns in the same period. But if he doesn't do his job perfectly, the patient may die just as dead as if the surgeon slips up. Cleaning here bears no resemblance to cleaning in an office building, where a missed coffee spill is just a stain on a carpet. If the

Main O.R.'s seamless gray terrazzo floors, made of marble chips in a poured, nonconductive, epoxy resin, aren't spotless, the patient may die. Similarly, if the undersides, as well as the tops, of the O.R. tables aren't perfectly disinfected, a patient may end up dead of what is called a "noscomial infection," an infection picked up in the hospital. Thus, what anesthesiologist Michael Myers says about his colleagues may be said with close to equal validity about the men who are just now removing the last of their equipment from Room 4: "It's a job, but there's always that subliminal pressure—knowing it's not quite a job. If you're a major league pitcher and you pitch .950, that's amazing. But if you're a cardiac surgeon, or an anesthesiologist, and ninety-five percent of your patients make it, that's not good enough."

"Are you finished?" anesthesiologist Ross Taff asks one of the environmental service workers as he rushes into Room 4.

"Just" is the reply, which Taff, quickly followed into the room by associate chairman of anesthesia Dominic Nardi and anesthesiologist Howard Wulfson, barely hears. As the three anesthesiologists rush to ready monitor lines and medications, they are joined by Lee McFee, chief of the monitor technicians, and perfusionist Rachel Goodman, who each begin frantically preparing equipment in the room.

The four hundred-pound, lead-shielded wooden door to the room bangs against the off-white tile wall, as it is shoved open and a gurney bearing seventy-three-year-old Peter Bass is wheeled into the room. Bass is almost invisible behind the screen of bodies surrounding the gurney: the transporter pushing the gurney; a fourth anesthesiologist, who is hand-bagging the patient; a monitor tech who is operating an intra-aortic balloon-assist device, a form of temporary, partial artificial heart; the radiologist who was doing a cardiac catheterization procedure on the patient when he suffered a cardiac arrest ten minutes ago in the cath lab downstairs; as well as three nurses. They are followed by four O.R. nurses who begin draping the operating and instrument tables and lay out all the instrument sets needed for a cardiac bypass procedure.

The clock on the wall reads 1:21, which makes that the official time inside O.R. 4 but may be up to ten minutes on either side of the time on the clocks in any of the other fifteen rooms. If the Main O.R. is a world unto itself, separated as it is from the rest of the hospital and the town beyond, it is a world with sixteen different time zones, the time in each established seemingly at random as the clocks are set and reset over the years according to dozens of different watches. Cardiac surgeon Roy Nelson hurries into the room, followed by three surgeon's assistants. Nelson goes straight to the balloon pump, which is doing the work of the patient's damaged left ventricle. He is quiet for a moment, examining the images on the monitor screen built into the machine. "Most of what he's got is balloon, guys," he says, meaning that the balloon, which is expanding and contracting in the aorta, the outlet of the patient's heart, is doing most of the work of the vital left side of the organ. "We've got to go. His own pressure is low." The cardiac surgeon leaves the room as quickly as he entered.

The patient lies on his back on the table, at this moment the direct or indirect focus of attention of eighteen medical professionals. He moans as surgeon's assistant Mark Olshaker inserts a urinary catheter, and Dom Nardi hooks up monitor lines to the arterial catheter already inserted down in the cath lab.

It is 1:27 P.M. Nelson, his dripping hands held in front of him, is scrubbed and back in the room. As circulating nurse Molly Neil holds out a paper surgical gown, the cardiac surgeon, who rushed to the Main O.R. from his nearby office in the hospital, stabs his arms into the sleeves and spins around so that Neil can tie the gown in the back. "Put the balloon on standby and let me know what pressure we have," he orders.

"One-fifteen," says Lee McFee, glancing at the monitoring equipment atop the anesthesia stand.

"Okay. We have a pressure," says Nelson, noting that the patient is doing a bit better than he was a few minutes ago. As Bass's chest and abdomen are being slathered in Betadine, surgeon's assistant Dolores Hardy has already begun removing a vein from the patient's leg to use as a substitute for blocked coronary arteries.

Four minutes have passed since Nelson returned to the room. "Rachel, how're we doing?" he calls to the perfusionist.

"All right. Getting there," she replies, tightening a filter into place in the pump circuit.

"We need to get him onto bypass, that's the main thing," Nelson tells her.

Three more minutes pass. "I need a blade," says Nelson, who, his surgeon's magnifying glasses already on, is helping drape the patient. Three minutes later the tile-walled room reverberates with the sound of a sternum saw chewing through bone.

"Heparin's in," Ross Taff tells him. When things calm down, Taff, one of the four anesthesiologists who spend the bulk of their time in Rooms 3 and 4, the heart rooms, will be the primary anesthesiologist on the case. Nelson swiftly places his stitches to hold back the skin at the edge of his incision and seals off bleeders with the electric cautery.

"The pump's ready," perfusionist Goodman tells the surgeon. It is 1:43 P.M.

"Molly, did John go get me those antibiotics I asked for?" Taff calls.

"They're on the way."

"Thank you."

It is 1:45 P.M. "Go on bypass," Nelson orders.

"Dr. Nelson, you okay up there?" asks McFee, who is operating the balloon pump.

"We're on bypass," the surgeon replies.

"Okay," says McFee, "I'm turning off this balloon then."
"You can turn it off," the surgeon tells him, "but we'll need it when we come back off bypass at the end."

"Roy, have you had a chance to look at the pictures," cardiologist Ed King asks, referring to the images of the patient's coronary arteries produced in the cath lab.

"No," says Nelson, who is examining the heart, "and there are certain things I'll need to know."

Thirty-five minutes have passed since patient and staff entered O.R. 4. In that time the room was set up, the patient was anesthetized and prepped for surgery, the surgeon, his assistants, and the scrub nurse all scrubbed and gowned, veins were stripped from the patient's calves for use in the bypass procedure, the heart-lung machine was set up, the patient's chest was opened, and he was put on the pump.

Under normal circumstances, it takes about forty-five minutes just to prepare the heart-lung machine for a case. In fact, in the normal course of an O.R. day, the preparations for a coronary artery bypass, from the premedication of the patient in the hallway to the first incision, can easily take between ninety minutes and two hours.

24

1:47 P.M. Next door, in Room 3, Peter Walker is pacing with one unit of donated whole blood tucked in his left armpit. "It's my blood warmer," he says. "It's safe. It's effective. It doesn't get air in the system. In the old days they'd have walk-in donors. Today, with all the required tests . . . That's another downside of the AIDS epidemic." Ironically, not three feet from where the anesthesiologist is walking back and forth, there is an FDA warning taped to the end of the heart-lung machine, unnoticed by those in the room:

> Recall Warning Alert #854, June 25:
> Red Blood Cells, Fresh Frozen Plasma. Units CB83711, CB83714, CB80007.
> Community Blood Bank of Southern New Jersey, including New Jersey, Pennsylvania, New York.
> Blood products testing repeatedly reactive for the antibody to the HIV type 1 were distributed.

By now Vinnie Parnell has reattached both the aorta and pulmonary artery of Baby Morrell, which entailed not only sewing those "major" arteries, the thickness of a pencil, but also grafting coronary arteries, more like a pencil lead, to ensure the heart muscle a proper blood supply. That involved working with 8-0 sutures, a surgical thread so fine, Parnell noted, that anything smaller would require the use of a surgical microscope.

"Well, Peter, we're done," Vinnie Parnell announces now, adding, "I hope. Bridget, we'll take some blood," he tells the perfusionist, who releases one of her clamps and allows blood to cross to the operating table and fill David Morrell's plum-size heart. Parnell watches carefully, sealing off as many of the bleeders as he can, but it is impossible to stop all the bleeding from so small a heart. When he is off the pump, the infant will be given drugs to increase his coagulation, which, Parnell and Walker hope, will stop the bleeding.

"Mary, will you scoot under the drape and check our rectal probe," Parnell says, sending the nurse to make sure the temperature probe is in place. "Let us know if you find any gerbils under there."

For the next hour, as the child's body temperature is slowly increased, the team will simply wait and watch the heart, assessing the state of the bleeding. And tease Mary Brian.

"Hey, Mary, can I use a butter substitute?" Parnell asks the nurse.

"God. I'm always getting yelled at—'Mary, put more butter in your vegetables! Mary, put more butter in your vegetables!' I don't eat anything I make. Butter! Butter! Cholesterol! More butter! Butter!"

"How long have you been up there now?" Parnell asks Brian, who, seven months ago, after ten years as a cardiac nurse, left nursing to enroll at the Culinary Institute of America in Hyde Park, New York. She is back at the hospital this week, earning money while she is on vacation from cooking school.

"I've been there since January. It's a two-year program. Then I can do a fellowship after that."

"In what, sauces?" Peter Walker asks, laughing.

"I may do a fellowship in fish," the nurse tells him, and then launches into a discussion of the more revolting aspects of sausage preparation.

"Good God! Is there anything good for you?" Walker asks.

"I really like making bread," Brian replies.

"Great," Parnell says, "maybe you can specialize in hamburger rolls." Then, changing his tone, he says to Walker, "You know, I have to give Mary credit, to go from something high-paying to something she really wants to do. Where are you going to work, Mary? Some posh Manhattan restaurant?"

"No. The Doral—where I'm going to do my internship—is going to open a spa in Colorado. I think I'd like to spend some time in Italy first, and then go out there when they open it up."

"You're not going to open a posh Manhattan restaurant so I'll always have a table?"

"No, I'd like to open a pastry shop," the thirty-four-year-old nurse replies, a plastic bag of bloody surgical sponges in her hands, "maybe work for two or three restaurants and have a little storefront. I really like breads. You know, it's weird, but coming back here is starting to make me feel squeamish."

25

2:03 P.M. Michael Setzen unties his surgical mask, peels off his latex gloves and tosses both in an O.R. trash can. Lillian Paskow, her neck swathed in an enormous mound of white cotton packing and bandages, is technically awake, although not at all alert. At this moment she is being half lifted, half slid, in a maneuver that over the years has destroyed the lower backs of countless thousands of nurses and anesthesiologists, from the table in Room 1A to a transport gurney for the trip to the Recovery Room. "Thank you, everybody, for some excellent help today," says Setzen, who with another procedure ahead of him this afternoon, hurries out of the O.R. and through the halls to the family waiting room, just outside the Main O.R.

"Everything went well, very well," the dark-haired surgeon says, beaming as he walks up to Lillian Paskow's husband and sister. Without even waiting for questions, he smooths his full mustache and continues:

"She's awake at this point. You'll be able to see her in a couple of hours. She'll have a big bandage, a tube in her throat, a tube in her nose, and there'll be a lot of wires and beeping in there in the Recovery Room. I know I told you seven hours, but it went a lot quicker than we thought."

Lillian Paskow's sister has tears in her eyes. "There's nothing I can really say," she tells the surgeon. "Thank God it worked out smoothly, like you say. It's a dramatic shock, from the first time we heard about it to now. It takes time to work things out."

"Are you glad she did it?" Setzen asks.

"Oh, yes. We didn't have any choice," says Paskow's husband. "Yesterday, at the house, I thought she was going to say she wasn't going to do it. But if she puts her mind to something, the esophagus [esophageal] speech? She'll master it. She'll do it. You tell her what to do, she'll do it. If she's cooking, you say, 'take a pinch,' but the book says a teaspoon? She'll do what the book says."

"Will she have a new problem?" the sister asks, apparently afraid to use the words "cancer," or "recurrence."

"No," Setzen tells her. "Once she heals, she'll have radiation treatment to make sure there are no cells left. But . . ."

Lillian Paskow's husband interrupts. "Whatever it was, it's all out? It hasn't spread?"

"No," Michael Setzen tells them, attempting to provide both the reassurance being sought and honesty, "it doesn't appear to have spread."

26

2:18 P.M. Anthony J. Tortolani, chairman of the Department of Surgery, is sitting down, something he does not like to do, in his spacious but simply decorated departmental office. At this moment he is cut off from the rest of the world by the staff in his outer office: administrative assistant Connie Fontana, who juggles the dual schedules he maintains as department chairman and a cardiac surgeon—a task akin to keeping five oranges in the air simultaneously; supervising secretary Janis Collado, who handles his correspondence; secretary Jeanmarie Delzotto; and Maude Martocci, the former head nurse in the Surgical Intensive Care Unit, now the coordinator of surgical services, his departmental eyes and ears.

Though he may at times be forced to sit by the demands of his job, by social convention, or by pure exhaustion, Tony Tortolani never sits still. His long, whippet-thin body is in constant motion, a knee jiggling rapidly up and down, as he scans the paperwork prepared for his signature and neatly arranged on the glass-covered top of his spare rosewood desk. Glancing at his watch he reaches for the phone and punches the intercom button. "Connie? Would you call over to Room 3 and see if Vinnie has an idea of when they'll be through in there?"

"Right away."

Tortolani had an aortic valve replacement scheduled to begin at 3:00 P.M. in Room 4, but the emergency bypass under way there is forcing him to wait for Room 3 to become available.

Connie Fontana sticks her head around the corner into Tortolani's office. "Dr. Parnell says he hopes to be out of the room by three-thirty."

"So we can't possibly start before four-thirty, quarter to five. Okay, thanks Connie," Tortolani says, returning to the paperwork he loathes.

Tortolani is quick to acknowledge that he can barely sit at his desk, "let alone sit and listen to people complain," which makes one wonder why he took on the chief's job. "I don't enjoy that part of it. I do that because it's my responsibility and I go to all those meetings. I took on the job because I knew what North Shore wanted to be, and I knew what it could be, and I knew what it was. And it bothered me that North Shore was not as good a hospital as it could be. I didn't think we were training residents as well as we could train them, and I knew that, if I did that, I could make it better. That was a way of paying back: people trained me and I should train other people better than I was trained. I hate the politics of it. I hate the meetings. I miss not spending more time in the operating room. But I do get a lot of gratification out of bringing in Ph.D.s, giving them seed money—this past year we got a million and a half dollars in NIH funds in the Department of Surgery at North Shore Hospital. That's our Ph.D.s and our bioengineers. I'm not doing the work, I'm not a lab person. But I enjoy helping to get that going. And I really love working with the residents." And he leans on the attendings, the 160 community-based surgeons who do the largest share of the work at North Shore, to do their share of residents training, because, says Tortolani, he has data to show that the very surgeon who may say he is too busy to teach is often the best teacher. "Each year we have the residents evaluate attending staff. We run it through a computer blind, just by residency year and whatnot. We compiled it for several years and then we asked whether resident rating of an attending has any validity. So we took our data and compared it to the physician's complication rate, mortality rate, number of operations, and teaching, which we looked at as attendance at Morbidity and Mortality and Grand Rounds. We looked at research as number of papers written per year. And then we took the cases and balanced them by difficulty, so a guy who did all hernias wasn't compared to a guy who did all aneurysms. Well, the surgeons who had the highest rating by the residents were the surgeons who had the lowest length of stay, did the most operations, had the least complications, had the least deaths, wrote the most papers, and went to the most conferences. So the best guys were the best across the board. So when someone says to me, 'I'm so busy operating I don't have time to teach,' or, 'I'm so busy teaching I don't have time to do research,' or, 'I'm so busy doing research I don't have time to operate,' I don't buy it. When they say, 'If you want to get something done, give it to the busiest guy,' it's true—at least in surgery."

While he clearly derives satisfaction from some parts of his chief's job, Tony Tortolani's real professional love is operating. "I love to know that no one could have done it better than I just did it, and that I just saved somebody's life: whether he knows it or not; whether anybody ever says thank you; whether anybody ever pays the bill. When you're bone-tired, and it's 11 o'clock at night and you know you did a tough case and a lot of other guys either wouldn't have done it or couldn't have done it—that high is unbelievable. You know you did something that really was worthwhile. You really helped somebody. And you know, most of the time people don't even really know what you're doing. They say, 'Oh, yeah, okay. You're gonna do a triple bypass? Okay.' And you're saying, 'We're gonna prolong your life, we're gonna prevent you from having . . .' 'Oh, well that's good.' But if you have left main [coronary artery] disease, or triple vessel disease in someone who already has a damaged left ventricle, you definitely prolong life, that's well proven. If you have people with unstable angina, and you can't open up that blockage with angioplasty, you prolong life when you operate. And that's what we do.

"Our cardiologists are pretty conservative," Tortolani says, "so we're not going to see the stuff that they can handle medically. They don't rush people off to surgery. So most of the stuff we do is triple bypass, or cases where you'd like to do a triple bypass but one of the arteries is too blocked off. I'm not saying you get that high after every single operation, but when you do, that feeling is just incredible." He pauses. "I can't say I knew that before I went into surgery. Also, I think that in cardiac surgery, as opposed to other specialties, you're always putting yourself on the line, because there's no buffers; if the patient doesn't do well the patient dies. You can't say, 'Well, I replaced the hip and there's still some pain, the patient's really okay, he just complains a lot.' You can't say, 'Well, I fixed that hernia,' and, six months later, when the hernia comes back, 'Well, the patient had bad tissue, we'll fix it again . . .'" He laughs disparagingly.

"The scrub sink is the key thing," Tortolani says. "When you start scrubbing, what you're thinking about, what's worrying you, if you're tired, if your back hurts, if you have a stomachache, if you have a headache, you don't feel anything. It's like a high . . . It's like another world, and you're that way until you're finished. And when you get there, you don't start saying, 'Oh my God! This is a disaster.' You're going, and there's nothing that can stop you, you're just gonna keep going until this patient is out of there. If I know that patient has a bad ventricle, or even if I get hit by something I didn't expect, I'm just gonna plow ahead. It's like you see a 290-pound defensive man in front of you and you've got to make a touchdown, you're just gonna go ahead. It's either you or him; there's no options. That doesn't mean there's never been a patient with a calcified aorta, or something that technically kept you from doing the operation. But short of that, I've never opened somebody up and thought, 'Oh my God, this is much worse than I expected: Stop.'"

In this age of runaway health care costs, many would argue that there comes a point at which social considerations and responsibility, rather than surgical skill and hubris, should govern the decision to operate. But Tortolani argues that "a life is a life, it's not my problem how much it costs society. But society, or the insurance companies, may be saying, 'We can't afford that. We can't afford $250,000 for an eighty-year-old person to live another two years.' We are beginning to face these things that we didn't face five or six or seven years ago. Society can't afford for doctors to do every single thing they can possibly do. We can do more for people than society can pay. It's not that they aren't willing to pay for it—they don't have the money. It's not that hospitals are making fortunes; hospitals are going out of business. Doctors are doing very well, but they've always done very well. The main reason to do these people is that they're there and we think we can help them. But people can't afford it. Even the open-heart procedure. Let's say a double valve and triple coronary costs $10,000, that's as much as anybody ever charges—the average open heart case is $5,000 or $6,000." Tortolani adds that his cardiac surgery group accepts what insurance pays for close to 50 percent of its patients and says that he doesn't allow the office staff to harass patients for payment. "We don't have a collection agency. But, quite honestly, at North Shore we don't see the poorest of the poor. Our idea of poor is somebody who doesn't have insurance. But we don't

see the people who go to Bellevue's Emergency Room, who
have to have a shower to get rid of the lice before you can
examine them.

"If you do a major procedure on eighty-two-year-old Mr.
Jones and he stays in the Intensive Care Unit for three
weeks and two more weeks in the hospital, and a month
in a nursing home before he can go home and live with
his wife, who's had a stroke, that's costing somebody literally hundreds of thousands of dollars. And I think people
are saying, 'That's great for Mr. Jones who's eighty-two to
live for two more years, but we're paying for it.' Mr. Jones
can't, he doesn't have $250,000, somebody else is paying
for that.

"But I have an underlying philosophy, which I got from
Frank Spencer when I trained under him at NYU: 'Whatever it takes to save a life, that's what you do.' There're no
rules, there's no nothing. You break down any door, you
drag anybody out you have to drag out. You are responsible
for this person's life. It's your responsibility, nothing
supersedes that: not your family, nothing. He lived that. I
don't mean to make him a God, but he lived it.

"There's the Greek ethic, that says you do what's best
for the majority of the society. Then you have the Jewish
ethic, which is, 'These are the rules and you follow the
rules.' Then there's the Christian ethic, that says what's
best for the weakest is what you do for everybody. I think
I was raised with that mentality, although I can't say my
mother told me this, or the priest told me this," says Tortolani, who attends mass every Sunday and goes to early
mass on days when he faces difficult decisions. "I believe
if you don't help the weakest, if we don't find the weakest
link in the chain and fix it, the chain is weak. That's what
worries me: our society tolerates poverty; our society tolerates people sleeping in the streets of New York. So I
don't think it's up to me to decide to give up on a patient.
My feeling is, when God decides, then there's nothing I
can do. Because I'm just fooling around."

Tony Tortolani doesn't seem so much to have chosen surgery as to have been called to it. "I can't say that it ever, ever bothered me to make an incision. I'm not the greatest surgeon that ever lived," Tortolani says. "I'm not the smartest guy that ever operated on somebody. But I would say that from an intern's first time he ever operated on somebody, if he stays in surgery, it probably never bothered him to make the incision. That's not a learned thing, because he'd never done it. It's something that he doesn't have a problem with. That's part of the makeup, it's what makes a guy go into it. I think it's a God-given ability, either you have it or you don't. It's your talent. And what I think— honest truth?—is that you have an obligation to fulfill that talent. People who take their surgical abilities and use them just to make money, or abuse them, that's the worst sin in the world. If my talent were mopping the floors, for instance, then that's my talent. That's what God put me on this earth to do, and that's what I'd do," says Tortolani, who operates about two hundred times a year.

There has been much written and said about the "surgeon's personality," which, like someone describing great art, or obscenity, Tortolani says he can't quite define, but knows it when he sees it. "I don't know how you say this, but people who do heart surgery are constantly proving to themselves that they're as good as their last operation. I think heart surgeons in general are people who constantly have to prove to themselves that they really are as good as they think they are, because nobody else knows. So there's a certain amount of insecurity in heart surgeons. It's that constant inner challenge. It's not outside, because it's so private: I mean, who knows what you're doing back there? I really believe the great heart surgeons in this country, the Spencers, the Shumways, the Eberts, if you get to know them, are very shy individuals. If you come up and talk to them, they'll talk to you, but they won't initiate conversation. They're almost painfully shy people.

"There's a drive that the cardiac guys have that's different from the other people. If you look at the number of heart surgeons who sit in the lounge, or who sit at their desks, or who sit back and take a day off, or the tennis players and the golfers, they're practically nonexistent. We all do as many patients as we can—no cardiac surgeon turns down a patient. Nobody says, 'Gee, I'm too tired, I'll let somebody else do it.' Most of us make a lot of money, so you don't have to do one more case because you need the money. It's not like somebody who does two hernias a week who's got to do his two hernias. Most cardiac surgeons live to work. Their biggest thing is they'll drive a fast car home at night, a Porsche or a Corvette or something. But they're not people who enjoy life the way you would think people enjoy life." At least not when they're trapped behind a desk, waiting for an O.R. to open up.

27

Tony Tortolani is the first to admit that those who knew him when he was growing up would have been hard-pressed to predict, "This guy's gonna be a heart surgeon someday" or "This guy's gonna be chairman of the Department of Surgery." "I got out of high school with an eighty average. I was a very modest student. There was nobody who told my folks, 'Your son is really smart, he should go to medical school.' When I was in junior high school, they told my parents I should get a trade and go into the navy. If my parents had ever listened to the advice all the teachers and guidance counselors gave them, none of their kids would have gone to college. We weren't supposed to be smart, we weren't college material. We were good athletes, we were nice boys, but maybe I should be a cop in town, or go to work with my dad," who made his living as a part-time country club bartender and by installing, maintaining, and owning the coin-operated washers and dryers in the basements of apartment buildings in suburban Westchester County, New York. "If my parents had ever listened to that crap . . . Not that there's anything wrong with that. But we never listened to it," Tortolani says.

Like a number of his colleagues, he says that, despite what the guidance counselors were telling him and his parents, he knew from an early age that he was going into medicine. And, unlike most of his fellow surgeons and physicians, he can point to a seminal childhood event that he believes fueled that desire. "The only thing I can figure is the fact that I had polio when I was seven. I was in the hospital the summer of 1950, the whole summer, paralyzed on my left side with polio. I did okay with it, but I think that left a mark, and ever since I was seven or eight years old I wanted to be a doctor. There was no vaccine then, there was really no treatment. They gave you shots of, penicillin I guess, they put you in whirlpool baths, they gave you physical therapy. And I had bulbar polio, the kind you were supposed to die from, but I didn't. I never was in an iron lung, but I wasn't allowed out of bed and I remember seeing kids in iron lungs and the next day the iron lungs would be empty. When you're six or seven years old, that's really frightening."

Ironically, one summer day in 1976, when he had finished his cardiac surgery fellowship at New York University Medical Center, Tortolani and his colleague George Reed together visited the hospital in Valhalla, New York, where Tortolani had been hospitalized as a child. Reed, who is now chief of cardiac surgery at New York Medical College, at Valhalla, and Tortolani walked through the area that had been the polio ward. "I visited exactly where my bed was," he recalls. "It was the eeriest thing. It was like going back in time. It was painted different, but it looked exactly the same."

After graduating from high school in Eastchester, on the other side of Long Island Sound from Manhasset and North Shore, Tortolani went to Fordham University, not because he decided it was the one college in the United States that was the place he should go. "My choices were Fordham or Manhattan because my dad wasn't paying for me to go away to college when he had two more boys to put through college," Tortolani says. "It wasn't like, we'll visit twenty-five colleges over the summer. Fordham was close, only twenty-five minutes away. I got in my car every day and took the train and went to school." But like many choices, or nonchoices, in the surgeon's life, it proved to be serendipitous.

"When I was a kid going to college, my uncle owned a bar down the street from where we lived. His father owned it before him, it was a pizza joint and a bar, a local tavern. There was a doctor who always went in there and drank, he drank too much," Tortolani says. Tortolani's uncle happened to tell the doctor that young Tony was interested in a career in medicine, and the physician offered to help. As Tortolani tells it, the physician, who was in private practice in Westchester County, magnanimously offered to write a letter that he said would get the future medical student a job at Memorial Hospital [now Memorial-Sloan Kettering Cancer Center], where the physician occasionally referred patients. "He was kind of drunk when he wrote the letter," Tortolani recalls with a laugh.

"So I went to Sloan Kettering. I said, 'I'm Tony Tortolani, I have a letter, I want a summer job.' The guy in personnel looks at the letter and he thinks I'm nuts. But I figure, I'm in. I'm just a kid. Some doctor gives you a letter, he says you have a job, you have a job. The guy said they really didn't hire people for the summer. I said, 'Well, I've got the letter here.' He said, 'Well, maybe you can work as a volunteer.' So I met this lady Ph.D., and the first summer I worked as a volunteer, in the lab, at Sloan Kettering, working with mice trying to find a cure for cancer—and I thought I was going to find a cure. And at night I'd work at the country club as a busboy. Once I was back in college I'd work with her after school and on vacations, and I worked with her all through school.

"But how did I get a job at Sloan Kettering? I got it because some drunken doctor wrote a letter that meant nothing but gave me the courage to go there and say, 'I want to work here.' Only a kid who's kind of naive and doesn't know very much can get away with something like that."

Tortolani applied to, and was accepted by, a number of middle-caliber medical schools, but ended up at George Washington University, in Washington, D.C. "My youngest brother had gotten into GW to play football, he was an excellent football player," Tortolani says. "My dad didn't want my youngest brother to go to school in Washington alone. So if I could go to medical school there he could go to college there. So we went together." As it turned out, the GW football team played its last game at the end of that 1966 season, and Tortolani's brother transferred to the University of Connecticut, leaving him behind for four years of medical education—and, as it turned out, the chance to meet the woman he would marry.

"Before medical school I really thought I'd do research in oncology," Tortolani recalls, "but in medical school I really loved surgery. It was just exciting for me. I tell students and residents all the time: the field you go into in medicine is not an intellectual decision; it's an emotional decision, it's where you're comfortable, what excites you, what you like to do. It's not 'What should I do?' Very few people say, 'This is where the need is' or 'This is where I can make money.' It's what excites you. That's how I chose surgery. Also, you know what your aptitudes are. I think if I had to be something like a psychiatrist, I wouldn't have been in medicine: I could not have sat there and listened to people talk crazy stuff to me all day long. Not that there isn't a need for that, but I couldn't sit there. As I've said, I can hardly sit at my desk, let alone sit and listen to people complain and reveal their true problems. Someone has to do that, but I just couldn't handle it."

In 1969 Tony Tortolani arrived at North Shore for his residency. "When I first came here they weren't doing heart surgery," he says. "They didn't do heart surgery until my third year. There was no distinct Surgical I.C.U., it was part of the Recovery Room. This was just a modest-size community hospital with a medical school affiliation." But one thing North Shore had, that most facilities lacked, was a John Mountain, a general surgeon, who had been at North Shore since its founding sixteen years earlier, with a vision of what the hospital could become and what needed to be done to get it there.

"We tried to seed this place with bright, well-trained individuals who would try to carry it on to each succeeding level," the eighty-three-year-old Mountain says today. "But if you train people for three, four, five years and then you keep them here, you've got problems. You have inbreeding. In three generations they lose their perspective on anything that's new, or on change. So anybody we've thought highly of, we've sent out for further training in some special area and then brought them back. Tony Tortolani is an example of that. He did his five years with us and then [after two years in the air force] we were able to get him placed with Dr. Frank Spencer, one of the world's leading cardiac surgeons, for further training in cardiac surgery, then he came back here to put some life in our cardiac surgical program, which was foundering, and he's now the chief of surgery."

In fact, Tortolani didn't want to return to North Shore after his fellowship in Spencer's program at NYU. "George Reed and I were planning to go to Valhalla, we were all set, and Dr. Mountain very much wanted me to come back to North Shore. I wasn't going to come back." But John Mountain convinced Frank Spencer that North Shore needed Tortolani, and Spencer told him to accept the job. "And when your boss says, 'That's the job for you,' you can't not do it. And that's how I ended up at North Shore." Tortolani says.

"It was a primary and secondary care facility when I came back to it. Mike Myers [an anesthesiologist], who was an intern under me at North Shore had come back from Yale. And he brought the impetus to modernize the care of the surgical patient. He really came back from Yale with the concept of hemodynamic monitoring, the pharmacological manipulation of the blood pressure, he brought that to North Shore, against tremendous opposition and tremendous struggle, because he was much smarter than everybody else. Peter Walker, coming from Harvard to NYU, brought that to NYU, because in that area, NYU wasn't much farther than North Shore when I first got to NYU. It was ahead, but not that much ahead. But Mike Myers really, truly, brought it to North Shore. Mike Myers can't get things done politically the way Peter can. But Mike's heart is in the right place, and he may well be the smartest person in the O.R. He was a tremendous help when I started doing heart surgery," Tortolani recalls. "He would come in with me in the middle of the night. I used to stay every night then. I'd call him and say, 'Mike, this patient's in trouble.' He'd come in at eleven o'clock or twelve o'clock at night and sit with me for two or three hours. He didn't get paid for that. But if I was worried, he'd come in. How do you pay somebody for that? That's a pretty dedicated guy, although he would never admit that.

"So when I got here," Tortolani continues, "that's kind of the way it was. The department was basically a couple of full-time people who were doing run-of-the-mill general surgery, and a pretty okay Anesthesia Department—and Mike Myers. Then I got back here and everybody expected to find me as the nice kid who left, whom everybody loved. But I was trained by Frank Spencer, which meant 'You stay with the patient until you die or the patient dies, but nobody leaves until somebody's dead.' You slept next to that patient, literally. For two years at NYU, I slept in the Recovery Room. I'd stay in that hospital four, five nights of the week and I slept in the Recovery Room next to the patient. And I wasn't the only one who did it. That's just what you did. That's what I knew. If you wanted to do heart surgery, you sleep with your patients. Dr. Spencer didn't say that, but that's what you did," Tortolani says of

NYU. "And there were a bunch of us there at that time who have had successful, or extremely successful, programs: Wayne Isom, who's chief of cardiac surgery at New York Hospital; Tony Acinapura became chief at St. Vincent's [in Manhattan]; George Reed is chief at Valhalla; and Joe Cunningham became chief at Downstate and Maimonides [in Brooklyn].

"Anyway, when I came back to North Shore, it was, 'Oh my God, this guy's a maniac, he's crazy,' " Tortolani continues, "but I was there by myself doing heart surgery, fresh out of residency, and a year after that Mike Hall joined me, and that's how we got going. And we lived there for years. But that's the only way you can do it. Several people before me had tried to get heart surgery going at North Shore and failed. I think part of the reason I was successful is other people had laid the groundwork, had tried and failed and tried and failed. And having Mike Myers there was a tremendous help. For instance, when we wanted to use intravenous nitroglycerine, the Department of Medicine was against it. Roy Nelson was with us, running the cardiovascular research laboratory. We knew it was important, knew it was good, but we couldn't get it. So Roy Nelson called up a drug company and said, 'We're doing research with IV nitroglycerine in dogs, but we need clinical quality intravenous nitroglycerine. Can you send it to us?' They said, 'Sure, Doc.' They sent us the stuff and we kept it like it was gold, locked in Roy Nelson's office, and we used it on our patients, before they ever used it up in the Cardiac Care Unit, because we knew it worked and we couldn't get the cardiologists to agree, so we just did it. The first time we used IV nitroglycerine intraoperatively, the hospital was still blocking us. Mike Myers took the nitroglycerine tablets, crushed them, mixed them with sterile saline solution, and injected them into the patient.

"The basic operations have not changed," Tortolani says. "What gets the sicker and sicker, and older and older patients through surgery, be it a hip replacement or anything else, is the monitoring and the work that the anesthesiologist does at the head of the table. And that's all a spin-off from them getting the open-heart patients through. That's really where it all comes from. It's the anesthesiologists that have really made the advances. If somebody dies on the table now, it's a *big* deal. You don't lose that patient a day or two after surgery, or even intraoperatively, like we did years ago. And with all these ways we have of taking the patients' blood and giving it back to them, it's saved us transfusions, and transfusion reactions, and that has saved us patients. If the patient's bleeding you suck the blood up, you clean the blood, you warm the blood—as fast as the patient's bleeding, we can give it back to them. You can't bleed to death anymore. Almost anybody."

One thing that can die in the Main O.R. is a surgeon's marriage, and while Tortolani's is one of the exceptional unions that have survived the nights on end in the I.C.U., it hasn't been easy. "It puts a tremendous strain on the marriage, on the husband and wife in residency," Tortolani says. "However, most of the people you're with are in the same situation, so it's almost like being in the army and living on base. The hardest thing for my wife, and she was really depressed for a couple of years, was when I went into practice. She had great hopes that it would get better—not get better financially, because we never talked about what we would do if we made a lot of money, because it never entered our minds—but the time . . . When I went into practice, it was worse. Because at least when you're a resident, when you're off-duty, there's another resident there. No one is going to call you back. But when you're in practice you always can go back. You can't say, 'It's the attending's patient,' or 'It's not my night on.' It's your patient. The patient says, 'You're my doctor.' That's very difficult for the family—to realize it's never going to get better.

"I decided that I would never have hobbies. I don't play golf. I don't play tennis. When I went home, when the kids were growing up, I would be with them. We'd play ball or whatever. When I was doing my residency, my wife, bless her soul, would make dinner for me and bring the little kids—and they were little—down to the cafeteria and they'd eat dinner with me. When I was in the air force and I was moonlighting so we could afford to buy the house, she would drive over an hour with the kids in this little jalopy car we had, to bring me dinner to some little hospital in the middle of Kansas, far away from the base so they didn't know I was moonlighting, because I would go there from Friday night at six o'clock and I would moonlight until Monday morning at five A.M., and then go to work at the hospital. I'd work in the emergency room for all those hours straight so that I would make money so that we could afford the mortgage payments when we went back to NYU. Then when I was at NYU, she would take the kids and drive into the city from Manhasset and bring me dinner in the O.R. lounge and the kids would be running around there and that's how I'd see the kids. When I was at NYU I would stay there most nights, and when I had a night off, if I didn't have to stay in the hospital and sleep in the Recovery Room, I would come home at three or four in the morning, wake up the kids, hug 'em, tell 'em I was there, talk to them for a minute, go to bed, sleep for two or three hours, get up at five or six o'clock in the morning, get back in the car and drive back to NYU and work there for three or four more days. And that's what we did. It was hard for my wife.

"You just do it. You don't think about it. It wasn't like I said, 'My God, this is impossible.' It was just what you did. You just did it."

"Every step along the way," Tortolani says, "we made the decision together, except the decision to come back to North Shore. Beth wanted to go to Northern Westchester, she wanted to go to Valhalla. She had already picked out a house. She didn't want to go back to Manhasset. She resents that to this day. But the good thing about Manhasset, when my kids were playing ball, I could leave the hospital, go see them play and go back. It wasn't like I was sneaking out, I could do it because it wasn't like going from the city out to the suburbs and back to the city again. So I could be there for a lot of their activities. But it was tough. A lot of us have broken marriages, the kids get all screwed up. But my wife raised the kids. I can't take any credit for them turning out as good as they did. They've been clean kids, without drug problems, and she raised them. I was there in the distance. I hope I was a good example as an individual. I know a little bit about sports, so that's what I shared with them." The couple's son, Justin, is an All-American lacrosse player at Princeton, and their daughter, Julie, skied competitively and ran track at the University of Vermont. "I played rugby in college," Tortolani says, "until my father came to a game and said, 'You're crazy! You can't play this! You're going to go to medical school and you're playing something like this? No more.' So, no more. I told the guys, 'I can't play rugby anymore, my father won't let me.' I was twenty years old. But that's the way it was. That's the way I was raised. Your father says yes, you do it. Your father says no, you don't do it. There were no questions, no discussion."

While his earnings as a cardiac surgeon and hospital chief of surgery clearly place him at the top of any chart of physician incomes, Tony and Beth Tortolani live simply, albeit very comfortably. They have a large, traditional, simple home in Manhasset, less than ten minutes from the Main O.R., and a thirty-acre farm in Delaware, at the head of the Chesapeake Bay. Beth Tortolani goes down to the farm by herself on Thursdays and Fridays, and either her husband takes the train down after work Friday, or she drives back for the weekend. "When I go down, generally every other weekend in the fall and winter, I'm not going down there to work, I just go down to read. Beth loves it, so she doesn't mind that I don't work [around the farm] there. I don't want to go down there and have visitors. I just want to go down there and be with her, we'll go out to dinner, go to a movie, and once in a while my folks will come down. Maybe two or three out of all the weekends in the year we'll have another couple come down with us. The kids will come down whenever they want.

"We don't have a lot of friends. The friends that I have are the friends I had before I became chief: one of the anesthesiologists, a surgeon I was a resident with, and one from my intern year. The main reason we're all pretty good friends is the women get along so well. Every couple of weeks we'll go out and have dinner together. Once in a while we'll vacation together. But otherwise, I kind of keep to myself because you can't socialize and then tell somebody, 'Hey, you're not doing a good job.'

"Being chief is isolating. I tried to learn from Frank Spencer. How would Frank Spencer handle this? Or Tom Shires [the chief at New York Hospital-Cornell Medical Center]. They stayed separate. I'm not at their level. I don't have the national and international reputations they have. But I think the principles they used are good principles. It's hard to be hard on your friends. To be fair to everybody you can't always be nice to everybody, because people take advantage of friendships and that stuff. I have my family, I have my close friends. I'm very family-oriented. I have my parents. I see my brothers a lot. We don't belong to any country clubs. We don't own a yacht. We don't play tennis every Thursday night.

"I think I'd be much friendlier with a lot more people if I was just one of the boys," Tortolani says. "But you can't be one of the boys and not be one of the boys at the same time. If I'm one of the boys, they'd say, 'I could really use that O.R. time at eight A.M. Hey, come on, we're friends.' And I don't want any part of that."

Tortolani's son is considering entering medicine, and that makes the surgeon reconsider what such a career is all about. "It's a great profession. You're doing some good for the world. You get tremendous personal satisfaction.

You can make a good living. And whatever the reality is for him in medicine, that's what it is for him. He's not going to know it was better or worse in his dad's day. He'll do fine, and nobody can take away the satisfaction. If you help somebody, you help them. The government can't take that away. Society can't take that away. No one can take that away. You'll never be unemployed. You'll always be able to work in an emergency room and sew up some kid's head or fix some old lady's broken ankle. And you'll know you helped somebody. In fact, you really can't not work if you want to work—there's a town, there's a country somewhere in the world, that needs you. And that's a good feeling you have. You can always say, 'North Shore, screw off! I'm going to Iowa and work in an emergency room, I don't have to put up with this crap anymore'—if you want to say that. When I graduated from medical school, I said, 'I am never ever going to work to make somebody else happy. I've passed all the tests, and I've written all the papers that I'm ever going to write for somebody else. If they don't like me as a resident, that's okay, I know I can have a job somewhere. So I always worked very hard, but I never worked very hard to make the boss happy. I worked very hard because that's what I wanted to do. You spend your life in premed and medical school proving to somebody that you know something. I don't have to do that anymore. Ever.''

28

2:20 P.M. Calm has been restored to Room 4. Where there were eighteen people working during the initial stages of the bypass crisis, there are now eight: the surgeon, two surgeon's assistants, an anesthesiologist, a perfusionist, scrub and circulating nurses, and a monitor tech. Anesthesiologist Ross Taff is finally catching up on his paperwork, one vessel has already been stitched in place in the heart, and surgeon's assistant Dolores Hardy is removing a second from the patient's left calf.

"Is this the better of the next two, or the worse of the next two?" Roy Nelson asks.

"The better."

"Okay. Give me a three-millimeter vein, really tiny, and see if you can get another one out."

"Got it," says Hardy, who moves up the table to assist Nelson.

When the patient was wheeled into the room, his circulation was being artificially maintained, with the left ventricular assist device, the balloon pump, doing the pumping work for the heart, and with drugs maintaining a passable blood pressure. "What you have is a time frame in which you can restore coronary blood flow," Nelson explains, "usually about thirty to forty minutes." If good blood flow can be restored to the muscle, the heart, in that period, the patient has a reasonable chance of recovery.

Nobody is putting odds on the patient's chances of surviving this operation, but it was eminently clear at 1:20, just sixty minutes ago, that there were only two options for Peter Bass: turn off the balloon pump and take him to the morgue; or rush him to Room 4 and attempt a triple coronary artery bypass. Thus far, the second option seems to have been the better choice. While the procedure is certainly not routine, with the balloon pump still ready to go at the foot of the operating table, the staff has settled into a routine. Now it seems as if the patient will at least live until the time comes to turn off the heart-lung machine at the end of the operation.

29

2:30 P.M. Other than the fact that the dark gray terrazzo floor and the pale greenish-white tile walls are the same, Room 1 bears little resemblance to the charnel house it was a few hours ago. This half-million-dollar surgeon's workshop—and that's just the price for the bare walls, the floor, the heating and cooling, the electrical and anesthesia gas lines—has been cleaned and restocked. All replaceable lines and tubes are long gone. The Gigli saw used to amputate Andre Fogarassi's leg is but a bizarre memory, sent back to the main sterilization room for cleaning and repacking for use on the next unfortunate. In place of the heavy, crude instruments used for amputations, two trays of delicate tools have been laid out for use during pediatric procedures involving the ears and throat.

Vascular surgeon Larry Scher has returned to his Great Neck office, and the room now belongs to Michael Setzen, whose second case of the day is a piece of his surgical bread and butter: after spending the morning in Room 1A doing the most demanding, complex type of surgery he ever does, he is now next door in Room 1, doing one of the simplest: a combination of myringotomy with tubes, tonsillectomy, and, if necessary, adenoidectomy.

The patient, who has just been anesthetized and intubated, is a three-year-old boy with Down's syndrome. "These parents know a lot, more than an anesthesiologist," Nalin Sudan says, laughing. "No, they do," he insists. He should know. In addition to being a board-certified anesthesiologist, Sudan is boarded in pediatrics. "They've been through cardiac surgery, they've been through the I.C.U. They look and they listen. They ask questions. But if you've taken care of him before"—as Sudan has—"they don't ask questions."

The first stage of the surgery, the myringotomy, or piercing of the eardrums to relieve fluid buildup, and insertion of minute drainage tubes to keep the middle ear area clear, is done under an operating microscope, set at twice normal magnification. Setzen makes a minute, three-millimeter incision, inserts an ear speculum, cleans out the ear, suctions out the fluid, makes a second incision and inserts a .045-inch diameter Silastic drainage tube in the left ear. The entire process takes two minutes and twenty seconds. "I don't want him to bleed at all," he explains, the cautery ready in case. "He needs the ear because he must hear better so that he can communicate with his family and his family can communicate with him," Setzen says of the retarded child. The fluid accumulation and repeated middle ear infections have, at least temporarily, reduced the child's ability to hear.

After repeating the process in the right ear, Setzen moves on to the throat. "The tonsils we do because he's having difficulty breathing," he explains. And, indeed, after the surgeon places a Crow-Davis mouthpiece, or spreader, in the child's mouth, the view down the little boy's throat makes it evident why he is having difficulty breathing: most of the space in his throat that should be his airway is taken up by two pinkish-white masses, his enlarged tonsils.

Using a needlelike blade on the Bovie cautery, over the course of twenty-six minutes Setzen cuts out the two tonsils, at the same time coagulating the incision line and all the minute blood vessels he has cut. Simply removing one of the tonsils quadruples the child's airway. With the second removed, the throat is not recognizable as the same obstructed passage it was prior to surgery. The tonsils removed, the surgeon decides to shrink the adenoids by cauterization, rather than remove them. "Okay," he announces at 3:01, "that's it, the whole operation. Let's go see his parents."

30

3:03 P.M. Vinnie Parnell is using the cautery to seal off the remaining bleeders along the edges of David Joseph Morrell's incision and then begins pulling the sternum back together with wire stitches. He has already closed all his interior incisions and is now finishing the last part of his work. After eight days of life outside the womb and four and one-half hours of having a surgical team cut and stitch, the infant has a normally functioning heart: the ventricle septal defect has been repaired, and his aorta and pulmonary artery have been disconnected from the heart and reattached over the proper valves. Now, if the stitches hold and the delicate tissues don't tear, David has a good chance of living until, like the greatest percentage of the population, he dies in his eighth decade of some form of cardiovascular disease—which will have nothing to do with what was done here today.

Peter Walker is altering the mixture of gases and drugs that the infant is receiving, bringing him closer to the edge of consciousness, when Rocky Rossi comes back into Room 3 with more administrative work for Walker. This time it's a question about changes in tomorrow's operating schedule, which Walker quickly deals with. As he answers Rossi's questions, Walker disconnects Baby Morrell from the respirator and begins hand-bagging the infant. "Where I trained, at Mass General, we didn't use ventilators for the little kiddos," Walker explains. "We almost always hand-bagged. My professor, John Ryan, used to say, 'A ventilator doesn't have a soul.' "

If there is anything that Peter Walker has accomplished since coming to North Shore University Hospital a decade ago, it is that he has given the Department of Anesthesia a soul, along with a degree of professionalism unequaled by virtually any community hospital, and not excelled by most major university teaching facilities. When Tony Tortolani convinced Walker to give up his position as chief of pediatric cardiac anesthesia at New York University Medical Center in 1981, Walker joined a coalition of two warring groups of anesthesiologists—with two billing agencies but no residents and no nurse anesthetists. Within a year he took over the department chairmanship—the understanding when he was hired—and today there are close to forty anesthesiologists, about half of whom were trained in anesthesia at either Harvard, Yale, Columbia, or Penn, plus almost twenty certified registered nurse anesthetists. "My sense was that what was needed was a cascade of first-round draft choices," Walker says, "so I said to people, 'Come work here. It's a great environment for young Turks, and you're a young Turk.' " What he did by recruiting his "young Turks" was create an unusual environment for surgeons to work in in what is technically a community hospital. While surgeons and anesthesiologists traditionally view each other with suspicion, and not a little scorn—hence the "blood-brain barrier" between their work areas—every one of a dozen surgeons asked to name the outstanding feature of North Shore, responded without hesitation, "The quality of anesthesia." One cardiac surgeon summed it up best when he described the contribution of anesthesia to surgery as the "tractor factor."

The surgeon explained: "Before tractors were well-balanced, farmers could only plow level fields without risking having the tractor roll over on them. As the tractors got better and better, the farmers could make use of steeper and steeper fields. Well, anesthesia is the tractor, the patient is the field, and we're the farmers. In the past ten years, as monitoring, drugs, and anesthesia techniques have improved, we've been able to operate on sicker and sicker patients." It's not that Peter Walker is responsible for these changes and innovations, but he is responsible for having brought them to North Shore on a departmental basis. Where before he took over the department there were a few anesthesiologists capable of working on the steepest hillsides, now there is a staff of them.

Quality, Walker contends, begets quality. "Coming to North Shore is a career choice. You don't come here to get your ticket punched and move on," says the ascetic-looking New Englander, out of St. Marks, Harvard, and Boston University Medical School. "You choose the institution, you choose the peer group."

Anesthesiologists also come to North Shore for money: the newest members of the group, who, like associates in law firms, are employees of the group for their first three to five years, earn in excess of $130,000 a year, which is more than the vast majority of anesthesiologists in the Harvard system earn. And once a physician becomes a partner in the group, his earnings quickly approach the obscene. But they are earned: unlike the situation in some community hospitals, where anesthesiologists work on a case-by-case basis, or in some medical centers, where they work a set number of hours, North Shore's anesthesiologists are assigned to rooms, rather than cases, on a daily basis. The workday begins at 7:00 A.M. and runs until the last scheduled case in the room is finished. Thus today, after coming in two hours early, Walker will stay in Room 3 until the aortic valve replacement, which has not yet even begun and may run a good six hours, is finished.

Additionally, Walker radically altered the payment system for anesthesia. Rather than deal with the intradepartment warfare over payment, Walker eliminated the concept of individual billing and, instead, established a single pot that is divided up based on the number of hours worked, instead of on how much each patient pays. And, rather than draw a large chairman's salary in addition to his medical earnings, or, on the other hand, be financially penalized for the fact that his duties as chairman take him out of the O.R. several days a week, Walker simply asked that he receive the average share paid in a given year, plus 10 percent.

As part of professionalizing the department, one of the first things Walker did when he took over was to hold a meeting and announce that the days of masked anonymity for anesthesiologists were gone for good: from that day hence, every anesthesiologist would be expected to visit each of his patients in their hospital room the afternoon or evening before surgery. The system became somewhat unwieldy as the department grew, so that, today, department members sometimes cover for each other, with one physician visiting the patients of his colleague who may be either tied up in surgery or off-duty on a given evening.

The spirit of Walker's act has remained, however. "No matter how sick a patient is, you can still take time for those little things that make them comfortable," Walker says. "I'm amazed at how, with some of my sickest patients, you can just do something like putting a pillow under their head. You'd be amazed at the number of people who come to the O.R. without a pillow, without anything to support their head, and they're elderly or whatever and their head is just cocked back and they're left in the hall and nobody even says hello. Or you can do such a simple thing as watching the way you undrape a woman to start an IV. There's no reason why you have to expose her. You can just very gently do this in such a way that you preserve her modesty."

31

3:20 P.M. General surgeon Dan Reiner, who before dawn was vainly attempting to wrestle a pile of swollen intestines back into a trauma patient's abdomen, is now performing a laparoscopic cholecystectomy, the removal of a gallbladder through a one-inch-wide incision in the patient's abdomen. He has already inflated the abdominal cavity, using a long needle and CO_2, to create internal working space, and he has inserted a fiber-optic scope, connected to a videocamera, through the first of the four one-inch incisions he made in forty-two-year-old Gail Whitman's abdomen.

Reiner has not been home in two days. As chief of the trauma service, he was called back to the hospital at eleven last night to work on the stabbing case that occupied Room 6 until after eight this morning. The surgeon never did succeed in fitting all the patient's bloated intestines back into his abdomen. He had to leave the abdominal incision open a few inches, with cotton packing providing a protective cover, until the swelling subsides enough in the next few days to allow a normal closure. Reiner, one of North Shore's five full-time general surgeons, then went on morning rounds, canceled his appointments until 1:00 P.M., and crashed for three hours in one of the disheveled beds in the surgical on-call room.

After inflating Gail Whitman's belly with carbon dioxide, Reiner, third-year resident Ralph Cohen, and first-year resident Alicia Blackwood stood clustered around the patient on the operating table, staring intently at a Sony Trinitron monitor on a stand near the head of the table. They watched what appeared to be a live television broadcast from inside a wet, whitish-pink cavern. Something was on the outside of the cavern, pushing down into the ceiling of the chamber. "Twist the instrument down," Reiner, continuing to watch the TV screen, told Cohen. "Press down, now lighten up—it's sharp." His warning was propitious. No sooner were the words out of his mouth than the razor-sharp end of a metal tube called a "Surgiport" broke through the roof of the cavern. One end of the Surgiport is a cutting blade, while the other end of the hollow tube is set into a square of plastic that steadies the instruments passed through the tube into the patient.

With four Surgiports in place and Blackwood operating the videocamera inserted in one of them, Reiner inserted a surgical stapler—shaped, like most of the other laparoscopic instruments, a bit like a stork's bill—through another port. He gave the residents a brief tour of the anatomical landscape, ending with the gallbladder, a sac-like organ, about three inches long, attached to the bed of the liver, from which it must be removed without damaging the liver. He then used parallel strips of staples to seal off major blood vessels supplying the gallbladder, much as, in a procedure where use of the staples was inappropriate, he might use stitches to tie off vessels above and below the point at which he planned to cut.

Now, peering intently at the monitor, Reiner begins to use the cautery to cut between his rows of staples. Eerily, the smoke of burning flesh, trapped inside the abdomen, rises, creating clouds and mist that envelop the landscape in the pink cavern. Reiner and Cohen alternately manipulate the cautery, microdissector, heavy grasper, irrigation and suction lines, and surgical stapler. In just a few moments the gallbladder, charred and alternately angry red and black in places, is cut free.

"Who was that Civil War surgeon who set the record for amputations—six seconds and four fingers off the first assistant? Six seconds, four fingers and a testicle," Reiner jokes.

"First assistant? Wait just a minute!" cries Cohen, laughing.

And the work goes on.

32

That Gail Whitman should travel over 750 miles for state-of-the-art surgical treatment of her gallstones is ironic for two reasons: first, she is extremely distrustful and dismissive of mainstream modern medicine, a believer instead in herbalism, acupuncture, and meditation; second, she lives in Canada, whose national health system is held up as a model by many of those who accurately diagnose the American health care system as terminally ill. But eight years of herbs, acupuncture, and positive thinking have failed to dissolve the painful gallstones, and after researching the subject, she has decided she wants a laparoscopic cholecystectomy, and the only surgeon in Halifax, Nova Scotia, to offer the procedure has done a total of twelve, and Gail Whitman doesn't want to be number thirteen on his learning curve. She says she could have had the procedure done in Montreal, but she would have had to wait six months for surgery there, and besides, if she was going to travel all that distance, she decided she might as well come to North Shore, which is near her parents' home.

"I started to have symptoms about eight years ago," she says, sitting in her parents' spacious living room. "I thought I'd eaten a rotten walnut. It felt as if a boxer had slugged me. The pain just wouldn't stop. No amount of aspirin, no heating pad, could make it go away. The next time it happened I ended up in the Emergency Room, in Halifax, but they made me wait so long that the pain went away. About seven years ago I was given an appointment with a surgeon," the small, intense, woman continues, "and I was given Demerol. I couldn't take it, though, because I'm a meditator, and the mind is really important to me." She was afraid the narcotic painkiller would make it difficult to meditate. "Besides," she says, "I was going to the surgeon for information, and he wasn't giving me information— he was telling me to have an operation."

"Basically," she says, "what I found out was there are Western people, with surgery, and Eastern people, with herbs. My alternative people, my acupuncturist and herbalist, said I hadn't tried enough to consider surgery then. I hadn't had an attack for a year, but I knew the stones were still there. It seemed that while Western doctors had nothing to say, alternative doctors had a lot to say." But no matter what it was that they said, the pain wouldn't stay away. So Whitman began seriously considering surgery.

She says she has two friends who have gone through gallbladder surgery: one had traditional surgery on an emergency basis, was in the hospital for seven days, and took a month to recover; the other had a laparoscopic cholecystectomy and barely knew she'd had surgery.

"So I went back to asking questions," Whitman says, finally deciding she'd "come home for this. My parents have a business, and they've always kept me on the business insurance, so money isn't a consideration.

"I am scared of going under general anesthesia," she says, "really scared. When I go under I'm going to try to stay really focused, to keep telling myself it isn't time to die. I've been under twice in my life, so it isn't that I haven't had experience in the hospital, but I keep reading these reports of people who've died."

33

3:47 P.M. "Could I have that big grasper we call Marie?" Dan Reiner asks, extending his left hand toward scrub nurse Mary DiPalo. At the mention of her name, circulating nurse Marie Mara, who often works with Reiner, glances up, shakes her head, and then resumes work on the nursing notes, refusing to take the surgeon's bait.

Reiner takes the instrument he has been handed—which, to the untrained eye, is no different from the other scissor-handled stork bills with which he is operating—and slides it through one of the inch-wide incisions, from which he has removed a Surgiport. He locks the grasper onto the neck of the gallbladder and tugs, attempting to draw it out of Gail Whitman's abdominal cavity through the incision. But he is attempting to force the proverbial camel through the equivalent of a needle's eye, and he must pause to slightly enlarge the incision. A gallstone is wedged in the neck of the gallbladder and, Reiner tells the residents, "A stone impacted in the neck is the worst. I'd rather do a hot [infected] gallbladder. After all those fine moves, we have to go through this kind of torture."

After using a suction line to suck as much material as possible from the gallbladder, Reiner manipulates "Marie" to position the neck of the gallbladder just below the incision he has enlarged. Now he uses small forceps to reach into the organ and remove the stones, which are the size and color of peas, one by one. As he makes a small pile of stones, coated with yellow bile, on a surgical sponge on the instrument table, Reiner notes, "They're huge. You could make a bracelet out of these."

It is 3:59. Reiner gives a final tug and pulls the gallbladder, emptied of stones, through a one-and-one-half-inch incision in Gail Whitman's abdomen. Now he closes the four small incisions, one in her navel, one about six inches above it, and two a few inches to the right of it, about three inches apart. She will remark, about ten days after surgery, that what used to be a major abdominal procedure has left her with what look like three faint cat scratches on her stomach.

As he works, Reiner entertains the residents with stories from his own training days. "We had a patient when I was chief resident at the VA who expired there of old age," he tells them as he and they stitch. "And the morning after he died, my attending got up and said we should observe a minute of silence, because Mr. Soandso had been admitted sixteen times, and eighty percent of the residents to come through the program had touched his skin."

The residents laugh, and Reiner applies a final, Band-Aid-size dressing to one of the incisions, and announces, "Done! Finis! One hour and twenty-six minutes: near record time."

34

4:17 P.M. Seventy-three-year-old Peter Bass is now just another high-risk "cabbage" patient. Roy Nelson has finished bypassing three of Bass's blocked coronary arteries and has just taken the patient off heart-lung bypass. If all continues to go well, in another forty-five minutes he will be on his way directly to the Surgical Intensive Care Unit on the second floor, just outside the doors to the Main O.R. At this moment, anesthesiologist Ross Taff and monitor tech Dawn Bennett are on their hands and knees, underneath the surgical table, looking for one of the electrocardiogram lines that is supposed to be running from Bass's chest to the EKG monitor built into the balloon pump unit standing by the foot of the operating table.

"I'm eight and one-half months pregnant and I'm crawling around on the floor? This is nuts," says Bennett, who is, indeed, huge, and looking very tired. One of fourteen nurses and techs who are pregnant this July, she is a believer in one of the Main O.R.'s current superstitions: "If you want to get pregnant, sit on the pump chair for twenty minutes a day." Besides being an incredibly comfortable freebie from a manufacturer of disposable filters and supplies for heart-lung machines—the chair has a small plaque on the back reading, BENTLEY LABORATORIES, INC. WE SUPPORT PERFUSIONISTS—the gray, armless, typing-style seat is this high-tech world's fertility totem. "It worked for me," Dawn Bennett insists.

35

4:20 P.M. Orthopedic surgeon Nicholas Sgaglione is injecting 100 cc's of saline and epinephrine into Allison Cooke's right knee. The epinephrine will reduce bleeding, and the fluid volume causes the knee to swell and dissects, or separates, the tissue planes beneath the surface. The seventeen-year-old high school athlete lying on the operating table in Room 10 has been reduced to a two-foot strip of Betadine-swabbed flesh, with all but her right leg, from just above the knee to midcalf, buried in blue surgical drapes. "When I was a resident, these patients went into casts for six weeks. In the last five years there's been a reduction in that type of surgery. Now we start to move them right away," Sgaglione tells first-year surgical resident Bob Stewart, who is joining orthopedic resident Mark Arnold in assisting Sgaglione in this anterior cruciate ligament repair.

The operation will take a good three hours. It involves first removing ligament and bone from the front of the knee and tibia to transplant in the interior of the knee in place of a vital torn ligament that maintains the joint's stability as it flexes. "We call this a 'patella smile,' " Sgaglione says, taking a scalpel and making a two-inch horizontal incision across the bottom of Cooke's knee. "It'll be hidden under the kneecap and she'll never see it. It's extremely cosmetic. You know, she's going to take for granted that you stabilize her knee," the surgeon tells the residents, "but she's going to really appreciate that you were meticulous in taking the graft." Sgaglione makes a second incision about three inches below the first, and slides a stainless steel template under the skin between the two incisions and outlines the template with blue dye.

Because Room 10 is one of the rooms principally used for orthopedics, some of the baseboard-to-ceiling wall cabinets make it look more like a machine shop than an operating room. ORTHOPEDIC POWER EQUIPMENT reads one piece of plastic labeling tape, and beneath it is a list of what the cabinet contains:

Maxi Driver × 2. Mini Driver. Wire Driver. AO Air Drill. Synthes Reamer. Micro Oscillating Saw. Stryker Battery Hip Pack. Stryker Battery Oscillating Saw. Hall Drill. Versi Power Reams. Versi Power Drills. Versi Power Reciprocating Saw. Versi Oscillating Saw.

In another cabinet are Lag Screws, Bone Screws, Ambi Plates, a Shoulder Tray, a knee Arthrotomy Tray, an Iliac Crest Bone Graft Tray, an Ace Fischer External Fixator Tray, and a Harrington Tray. All that seems to be missing is the Mr. Goodwrench Tray.

Having marked his graft, Sgaglione uses the orthopedic equivalent of a saber saw to cut a small plug of bone loose from the middle of the bottom of the kneecap. He drills a hole in the plug, which is still attached to a strip of the patellar ligament, and runs a heavy blue suture through the hole, leaving the blue thread dangling out through the smile in the knee. Then he repeats the process where the ligament joins the tibia, ending up with a piece of ligament, about three inches long, with bone plugs at each end. He explains to first-year resident Bob Stewart that, when the sides of the patellar ligament are drawn inward and stitched together, the missing vertical section will not cause the patient any problems. He also tells Stewart that he's "going to get yelled at on that next rotation if you don't always have two instruments in your hands."

"Yeah, always hold the suction," adds Mark Arnold. "That way they can't give you the retractor."

"I've always wondered," Arnold says to Sgaglione, changing the subject, "what do we do if we drop the graft? Pick it up and use it, or harvest a new one?"

"That came up at a national meeting I attended," Sgaglione tells him, "and a famous orthopedic surgeon from Birmingham was honest enough to get up and say it had happened to him. He picked it up, washed it with Betadine, and used it." He pauses, and then concludes, "Of course, that's fine for Birmingham, but you couldn't do that here."

36

5:05 P.M. Given the choice, no one would be in Room 9 at this moment: not the patient, seventy-six-year-old Kurt Werner, who is unconscious, on his back, his feet up in stirrups; not colorectal surgeons Michael Moseson and Bart Hoexter; not surgical chief resident Jim Sullivan, or the two junior residents; not anesthesiologist Howard Wulfson; and neither scrub nurse Marie Delgato nor circulating nurse Beth Kane. Werner has recurrent carcinoma of the rectum and, as Hoexter told the two junior residents an hour ago at the start of the procedure, "This is the most aggressive operation anyone does for colorectal cancer. We already excised it locally and, despite radiation, it's back. So today we do the operation we least like to do. It's a much more aggressive situation this time. The cancer appears to be much deeper. It hasn't metastasized yet so we want to use this golden window of time to get it out."

The surgeons plan to remove the patient's anus, rectum, and the lower two to three feet of his large intestine, with Hoexter working up from below, and Moseson eviscerating down, from above. It is a savage, bloody, and disfiguring procedure, so much so that Howard Wulfson comments: "You hang around the O.R. long enough, you hear a lot of gallows humor, and you realize that the world is not a fair place. Bad things happen to good people. But this?" He shakes his head. "My wife wonders why I often come home exhausted and demoralized."

The work began with a urologist inserting red and blue catheters in Werner's ureters, red on the right and blue on the left. That way, if the ureters are cut during the procedure, they can be properly reconnected by simply checking the color of the catheters. It would not be surprising if they were accidentally cut, given the bloodiness of the procedure and the amount of cutting involved. Knowing that he would lose a great deal of blood during surgery, over the past month the patient made an autologous blood donation, arranging to have two units of his own blood stored for use during surgery, thus reducing his need to rely on possibly HIV-contaminated donated blood.

Hoexter began the procedure by making a ten-inch vertical incision down the midline of the patient's abdomen, and then extended it lower by cutting around the bellybutton. "The liver feels clean," he announced, after palpating it, searching for cancer that may have spread from Werner's colon. "The CAT scan does give you a good picture of the interior of the liver, but look and feel are still the best way to check the surface," he told the two second-year residents, who were working with him in the abdomen. But he kept checking. If the cancer had spread to the liver, the operation would be over. Hoexter would close and Werner would be told that, in effect, all modern medicine could do for him is attempt to make him comfortable as the malignant cells run rampant through his body and system after system collapses, until he dies.

Moseson and Sullivan, who have each been involved in other procedures, entered the room while Hoexter was finishing his inspection of the liver. Hoexter looked up as he finished and said, "Mike, the liver's clean."

"Liver's clean? Good. Then I can start." Moseson replaced Hoexter in the patient's abdomen, and Hoexter and Sullivan began their work at the lower end of the table. But just as they did, circulator Beth Kane, whom a clerk had just handed two units of whole blood, finished reading warning labels on the bag and asked, "What's HBsAg? That's not AIDS, right?" At the uttering of the word "AIDS," work stopped and the room fell still.

"No. That would say HIV-positive," someone immediately responded. But no one was able to translate the acronym correctly. They knew that the symbols meant that Werner was infected with type-B hepatitis virus. But was his blood infectious, and therefore a threat to the surgical staff? Hoexter, who had not yet begun cutting, but was scrubbed, broke scrub by taking one of the units and heading out into the Main O.R. to discover what unpleasant surprise the staff in Room 9 had just received.

Now, a few moments later, Hoexter, with his rescrubbed hands in the air, shoves his way back through the door of the room and announces, "That's surface antigen positive. He's infectious."

"I'd like goggles please," says Moseson, stepping back from the table. "Everybody double glove." Moseson and the two junior residents have been vaccinated against hepatitis B.

"Shit," mutters Sullivan, who has not bothered to be immunized. "I'm an idiot. I want a size eight," he announces to Kane, holding out his already gloved hands for an additional pair.

37

5:15 P.M. Room 4 looks as if a bloody hurricane has roared through it. Discarded monitor lines, tubing, and blood-soaked surgical drapes and towels litter the floor. And Peter Bass, who is just now being slid from operating table to transport gurney, looks as if he didn't heed the warning to leave the room before the storm struck: he has a long row of surgical staples down the center of his frail chest; clear drainage tubes are carrying pinkish fluid to Hemovac drainage units lying beside him; there are drains in both his legs; his body is crisscrossed with colored wire EKG lines; another set of lines leads from his subclavian artery to the balloon pump at the foot of the bed; and he has an oxygen mask over his face and is being hand-bagged.

But he is leaving Room 4 alive, which is saying a great deal, given that he entered it that way only with the help of mechanical and electronic supports.

On the other side of the sterilization, lab, and storage space that connects Rooms 4 and 3, Peter Walker has completed almost an hour of preparation and is just finishing putting Lydia Slatalla to sleep for the replacement of her failing aortic valve. As he checks all her lines for a final time before surgery, he consults with another anesthesiologist, who objects to doing one of tomorrow's cases. The patient is scheduled for a simple vascular procedure in one of the eight O.R.s in North Shore's free-standing ambulatory care center. However, anesthesiologist Alan Rachleff tells Walker, while the operation couldn't be simpler, the patient is a man in his 60s who has already had one heart attack and has a number of other medical complications. "I don't see a lot of grays," says Rachleff. "I see blacks and whites, and this one is black. I see this as a full-blown, tough case. We bring him down here to the Main O.R. and we do him right. And we do him alone. I won't do another case," he says, referring to the practice for some simpler cases of having an anesthesiologist—a physician—cover two rooms at once, with certified registered nurse anesthetists—nurses with specialized training in anesthesia— actually anesthetizing the patients.

"Let me look at the chart later and I'll see what I can do," Walker tells him.

"Karla, we'll probably use the St. Jude's valve," Tony Tortolani tells circulating nurse Karla Nash. "If it doesn't work, we'll use a pig valve."

"You're using mechanical valves?" the nurse asks, knowing Tortolani's preference for the natural pig valve.

"With someone in their sixties, we may save them a second operation," he says, explaining that, while the use of the pig valve does not require that the patient always take a blood-thinning drug to prevent clotting, the pig valve would have to be replaced in about ten to twelve years. On the other hand, although the pyrolytic carbon mechanical valve does require that the patient always take an anticlotting agent, and although the patient may be aware of a barely audible "click" each time the mechanical valve opens and closes, it should last for fifteen to twenty years. Thus, a patient being given a valve at sixty is better off with the mechanical device because she is unlikely to live long enough to need it replaced in another open-heart operation.

Lydia Slatalla is, in fact, just sixty. She has been hospitalized a number of times—for a tonsillectomy as a child, an appendectomy at nineteen, a hysterectomy in her thirties, kidney stones in her forties and the removal of a leg tumor in her fifties. But until she began to experience acute shortness of breath about two months ago, she had never had an indication that she might have heart disease—which is surprising, given that her father died of a heart attack at thirty-nine and her brother died of one at thirty-seven. "Did you know her son was just catheterized?" Tortolani asks Walker. "He's coming in in about a month for us to fix his heart. Talk about bad genes."

38

5:30 P.M. "This is a virgin knee, which should be clean
. . . and it is," Nick Sgaglione announces, clearly pleased
with what he sees on the Sony Trinitron monitor in Room
10. Now that the bone and ligament graft has been initially
prepared for implantation in Allison Cooke's right knee,
the arthroscopic portion of the procedure is getting under
way.

Sgaglione and the residents have made three small incisions, similar to those made during the laparoscopic gallbladder operation, one at the top of the knee and one on
each side of the bottom, for the placement of three ports:
one for the arthroscope, linked to a videocamera; one for
instruments and tools; and one for the fluid line, to keep
the knee filled with the saline solution that separates the
tissue planes in the joint. The tattered ends of the patient's
torn anterior, or front, cruciate ligament flutter in the liquid. Viewed through the liquid, the cartilage that serves as
the joint's cushion looks like a white rubber shower mat.

The surgeon trims away the remnants of the torn ligament to improve the view, and then uses the arthroscopic
motorized shaver, with its spinning cutting blade, to bite
through the tissue and reach the bone at the top of the

inside of the joint. Then he replaces the blade with a burr, and bores a hole in the bone. As Sgaglione works, circulating nurse Sue Burke, who went to art school for a year, remarks that she views the surgeon as "an artist with a canvas. All they see is what's on the canvas and right in front of them. They just see the project. And, like the artist, they have certain materials, and a certain amount of time in which to work.

"It's amazing, the changes in here. Ten years ago I'd watch them do this and they'd make big cuts on both sides of the knee and then feel around, bend the knee, feel in there and say, 'That's loose,' or 'That feels better.' "

"You play golf?" Sgaglione asks the orthopedic resident.

"Yes," Mark Arnold replies. "We went up to Vermont for a weekend and took some lessons."

But Sgaglione doesn't appear to be listening. Instead, he points to the view on the monitor of the top of the anterior of the knee and says, "We're going to put a graft in there. It's like tacking something to the ceiling."

39

5:55 P.M. There is no way to know at this moment whether Kurt Werner ever paused during his seventy-six years to consider the subject of animal rights and medical experimentation on animals. But whatever feelings he might have about the issue, he is now benefiting from the sacrifice of countless thousands of animals.

Both Michael Moseson, working in the abdominal cavity, and Bart Hoexter, working in the anal area, are using surgical cutter-stapler combination instruments that speed the operation and reduce the chances of injury caused by a misplaced or missed stitch—instruments perfected and tested on animals. Moseson is in the process of severing the lower three feet of Werner's colon. Rather than tie and sew it above and below the point at which he needs to cut, Moseson places one part of a two-piece stapler below the organ and another piece directly above it. The two parts of the stapler are then locked in place, and as Moseson pulls the trigger of the pistol-shaped plastic device, it simultaneously lays two lines of stainless steel staples across the colon and cuts between them with a built-in knife blade.

Hoexter, who has already sutured the anus closed, is carving an ellipsoid around it. There is, unfortunately, no other way to properly describe this horrific procedure than to say that he is coring Werner as one might core an apple. Like Moseson, Hoexter is aided in this work by a surgical stapler, this one an Ethicon Proximate Linear Cutter. Unlike the GIA, this is a narrow one-piece device that lays down a single row of staples and cuts along the line at the same time.

It is 6:00 P.M. The few unbloodied patches on a pair of stainless steel forceps sparkle as the instrument, shoved down from above by Michael Moseson, emerges into the bright O.R. light shining down between the patient's legs. Jim Sullivan grabs the cloth umbilical tie locked in the teeth of the forceps and gives it a hard pull, drawing the last three feet of Kurt Werner's colon and rectum down the gory carved passage through his pelvis. The arms and chest of Sullivan's blue paper surgical gown are soaked in blood as he finishes cutting the anus free and delivers the three-foot-long, cancer-riddled specimen.

40

6:05 P.M. "There's the valve, Peter. Not good."

"Real rock pile?"

"Real rock pile," Tony Tortolani tells Peter Walker. Examining Lydia Slatalla's severely calcified aorta, Tortolani is surprised not that the woman was experiencing the symptoms she was, but that she lived until she was sixty without experiencing them. Slatalla is now on the pump, and the temperature of her heart has been lowered to 47 degrees Fahrenheit, to protect it while Tortolani works. "How much does she weigh?" he asks.

"One hundred and seventy pounds," Walker tells him. The anesthesiologist has made it a point to know the patient's weight because that number is used to calculate all his drug dosages.

"There's no end to this," says the frustrated surgeon, cutting away more of the calcification. "Let me have a St. Jude's measure, a 21."

"A 21?" repeats scrub nurse Janice Burke.

"Yeah. And you'd better give me a 19, too."

Burke opens the blue, molded plastic case holding the Model 903 St. Jude Medical Mechanical Valve Sizer Set and takes out the 19- and 21-millimeter clear plastic sizing rings. She hands Tortolani the size 19 ring, attached to its holder, and he places it in the aorta where the valve will be seated. Then he tries the 21. "Nineteen it is," he tells Burke.

"How did your meeting go today, Peter?" Tortolani asks, as he trims away the last of the calcium deposits in the aorta.

"I was tied up with Vinnie's transposition. Dom had to take the meeting for me. I haven't talked to him yet. How about yours?"

"I hope Dom had a better time at your meeting than I did at mine." The two unlikely allies, Anthony Joseph Tortolani, second-generation Italian American, first person in his family to go to college, and Peter Fitz-Randolph Walker, one of the last of the noblesse-oblige WASPs, exchange a knowing laugh.

As Tortolani explains it—and Walker says virtually the same thing using similar language—"Peter and I knew one another at NYU. He lived in Huntington. Then I got word that Peter was tired of commuting, his kids were starting to grow up. Well, the chief we had was an older man who'd kind of inherited the position. Mike Myers was the heir apparent. He's a brilliant anesthesiologist, but wasn't the right person to deal with the politics involved. So I brought Peter out, and as soon as everybody met him, they said, 'He's got to be the next chief.' So he was out here about a year and the older fellow retired—he wasn't forced out— and Peter became chief. Peter and I are not close in any social way, but we're very close professionally. We think the same. If you say to me, 'What's Peter going to do in this situation?' I'm going to know. And Peter will know what I'm going to do. I have great respect for Peter as a physician. He has tremendous empathy, tremendous concern. He doesn't distance himself as far from the patients as I do. He never makes mistakes. He never has a bad day. He never lets the surgeon down. He's always absolutely alert. He's extremely bright. I don't think he's as innovative as one or two of the other anesthesiologists are. I don't think he soars as high as they soar—but he never crashes. They don't crash either, but they can worry me at times." Tortolani laughs. "Peter never worries me. They can be distracted. Peter is never distracted. When he gets in the operating room, he's not thinking about politics, or some other anesthesiologist, or some surgeon.

"When we go to meetings, Peter will talk a lot," Tortolani says. "He usually has a whole lot to say. I don't have a lot to say. I'm happy to be as involved as they need me to be. But my feeling is, if Anesthesia's got a problem, I've got Peter Walker. I don't want to run Medicine, I don't want to run Pediatrics. But keep your hands off Surgery, because I'll break 'em if you get too close. I'll help you, and if I need help, I'm going to ask you. But keep off my turf. This is my turf, I'll take care of it. So Peter and I are different that way. But he's a very good friend. If I said, 'Peter, can you help me?' I know he'd say yes, and he would mean it and he would do it.

"In the Main O.R. there are probably two anesthesiologists who aren't up to par," Tortolani says. "What Peter does is make sure they do cases that they're competent to do. He's not going to put them on a baby's cleft lip, he's going to put them on cases where they're not going to get into trouble. They're not dangerous guys, but you wouldn't want them on the ruptured aneurysm in a ninety-seven-year-old lady. I'm not being critical, because there're also surgeons I wouldn't allow to do certain cases. If they brought a case in I might say, 'Listen, you can do that, but if you're going to do it, have somebody else do it with you, or for you,' or 'I want Dr. So-and-so to consult on this case, and I want the family to know that Dr. So-and-so may be in the O.R. and may be involved.' It doesn't happen often, because most of the guys know the rules and don't want trouble."

41

6:16 P.M. The inside of Allison Cooke's knee looks like an ice floe after a seal kill, with bloody bits of tissue and bone shavings despoiling the wet, white, silent world. An enormous screw looms on the video screen, wobbling from side to side as Nick Sgaglione works to manipulate it into the hole he has drilled in the top of the inside of the seventeen-year-old's knee.

The surgeon has already used his arthroscopic instruments and the scope to position one of the bone grafts into the hole. He is now attempting to screw an "interference fit screw" into the hole with the graft, wedging the bone permanently into place. Sgaglione strains to get the screw in, but it just won't fit. So he backs it out and tries again with a slightly smaller screw, which slips from the instrument's grip. After fishing about with a grasper, Sgaglione finally retrieves the screw and gets it into the hole. Now he bends Cooke's knee to make sure that the free end of the graft isn't trapped in the joint. It isn't.

"I need a DePuy Kurasaka screw, twenty-one millimeters long and nine millimeters wide," Sgaglione tells circulating nurse Sue Burke, as he drills the channel for the piece of bone at the lower end of the graft. With the hole completed,

Sgaglione repeats the process he went through to place the bone plug in the top of the knee. This time, however, in addition to using the interference fit screw to hold the graft, the surgeon adds two heavy sutures, running through a hole in the bone graft, which he screws to the top of the tibia using a second screw and a washer. Thus the bottom of the graft is doubly anchored. "It takes five minutes extra to do this now," he tells the residents, "and this girl's going to come to me for the rest of her life, any time she needs an orthopedic surgeon."

It is 6:40 and Sgaglione and the residents have completed suturing their incisions and have bandaged the knee. The leg is then put in a Bledsoe Brace, which makes it impossible for it to move laterally, but allows the joint to flex. And the joint will be flexed, and flexed, and flexed, even before Allison Cooke is out of bed. A continuous passive motion, or CPM, machine is placed beside her on the gurney, and her leg will be strapped onto it as soon as she reaches the recovery room. The CPM machine automatically and continuously raises and lowers the leg, without pausing, bending the joint and straightening it out.

Tomorrow, if all goes well, Allison Cooke will go home. She will wear the brace, and use crutches, for one month, and will suffer the torment of physical therapy for three to six months. But in the end, despite suffering what without surgery would be a crippling injury, she will return to athletic competition.

42

6:47 P.M. The surgery in Room 9 has just resumed, following a five-minute break dictated by Kurt Werner's substantial bleeding and his need for a transfusion. In addition to the unit of his own blood and the saline solution he was given earlier, he has now been given an additional unit of Hespan, a volume expander to reduce the amount of additional blood needed, a liter of saline, the second unit of his own blood, and two units of donated blood. It is an irony lost on no one in the room that the odds are overwhelming that the donated blood Werner so fears will be purer than his own hepatitis B-infected cells.

While similes involving food and food preparation may seem out of place in discussions of brutal, disfiguring surgery, it is difficult not to think of a Thanksgiving turkey as Bart Hoexter and Jim Sullivan are completing the closure of the gaping wound between Werner's legs. Where there was the opening of a natural body cavity, now there is only a row of heavy sutures. Mike Moseson and the junior resident have replaced Werner's rectum and anus by creating a stoma, or opening, in the side of his lower abdomen. They have drawn the new end of his colon through the opening and turned back the edges, creating a round, puckered lip of tissue. This is where Werner will attach the ostomy bag, the device he will use to make up for the loss of his rectum and anus, when the freshly wounded tissue heals.

"So what did we learn today, boys?" Moseson asks the residents.

"That radiation stinks," the blood-soaked Sullivan pipes up, thinking of the failure of the earlier, less radical attempt to cure the patient.

"That ripping someone's rectum out is not appealing surgery," Moseson says, answering his own question, "but there isn't an alternative at this point, unfortunately. This is still the gold standard."

43

7 P.M. Other than the drastic reduction in activity and
staff, there is nothing in the isolated world of the Main
O.R. to indicate that, in the world beyond, this summer
day has slid quietly into twilight. There are no windows to
admit the orange glow of quickly fading sun, now hovering
close to the Manhattan skyline to the west. The temperature in the rooms varies between the low sixties and sev-
enties, depending upon where the last surgeon to work in
each of the rooms left its thermostat set. Whatever the
temperature, the rooms are still a good fifteen degrees
cooler than the outside environment. And, with the air
prefiltered in the hospital's central heating and cooling
system, and refiltered before it enters each room, a scant
seven percent of the particulate matter that enters lungs
outside the building reaches them in the rooms here.

It wasn't like this fifty-four years ago, when John Mountain, who at age eighty-three still comes to his office in
North Shore's Department of Surgery seven days a week,
was training in the city. Mountain, who has never held the
title of chief of surgery at North Shore—because he never
wanted it—has shaped the department and the entire hos-

pital with his power of persuasion and his behind-the-scenes political acumen. He is the hospital's institutional memory and can recall an earlier era, prior to the 1953 opening of North Shore, in which air conditioning did not exist in the O.R. "Windows were open, the street dust came in. Fans were on, you wore street shoes without covers. I often wondered how we survived, but we did. It was bad enough on the personnel, you became inured to it. But in the heat of the summer, with the patient under this myriad of drapes and blankets being given anesthesia—and early on a great deal of it was open-drop ether—if the temperature in the room was one hundred, which it probably was, it must have been well over one hundred underneath all the drapes and the lights."

Even in the dead of winter, with the windows shut, those in the O.R. were aware of the outside world, Mountain says, recalling one particular late winter night in 1936 or 1937: "The operating room was on the sixth floor, and one of New York's great surgeons was doing a procedure under local anesthesia on an elderly lady. Light reflecting on snow coming down made it very bright out, and for a split second I could see a reflection in the mirror of one of the overhead lights of what looked like a wraith going down past the window. The woman screamed out, 'My God! I'm in heaven!' What had happened was somebody had gone out the window from a floor above. We looked around, and everybody was pretty stunned—the patient was wide awake, of course—and they asked the telephone operator to check the floors. Sure enough, somebody did go out a window and landed on the overhang over the ambulance area, which probably had three or four feet of snow on it. The snow saved the woman who had jumped, because she got some minor fractures and that was it."

While the environmental isolation of today's O.R. is striking visually, and probably in terms of its psychological impact on the staff, it is one of the more minor changes

Mountain has observed over the extraordinary length of his career. For instance, he says, "We didn't have any recovery rooms back then. The patient went from the room to the O.R. and back to the room, with or without special nurses. So if there were no recovery rooms, there were no intensive care units. All the care was given on the floors. Even when they began to have recovery rooms, they were closed at four or five o'clock in the afternoon. And even when they were open, you used to have to use considerable pressure to have the hospital muster enough help to keep somebody in the Recovery Room overnight. They'd usually make provisions for a few hours for an extremely ill patient, but they just wouldn't staff 'em. But a lot of patients seemed to survive.

"In those early years we very often gave fluid under the skin rather than intravenously. We didn't know anything about electrolytes, we didn't know anything about the physiology of respiration. We didn't have endotracheal intubation. We used to do many of our long cases under spinal anesthesia, which very often the surgeons would administer themselves, because we didn't have trained anesthesiologists at that time. I worked with one man on a long case, and if he was going to operate, I'd give the spinal, and vice versa. Somehow we muddled through.

"The surgery of the chest at that time was the surgery of tuberculosis. In my early days I worked one day a week at what was then known as the Brooklyn Home for Consumptives," Mountain recalls. "I used to go down and help a chest surgeon. I'd do general surgery all morning and then go down Tuesday afternoons and they'd do two operations that are not even done anymore. These were bloody operations on very sick people, in which you'd take part of the rib cage out to collapse the lungs. This was before the advent of the antituberculosis drugs.

"Anesthesia has been a major force in allowing us to carry these very ill people through very long and arduous and difficult procedures. Not only have the anesthesiologists developed the technical expertise, but there's a multiplicity of drugs that have come along that allow these people to get off the table with dry lungs and rapid recovery from anesthesia. These patients in the early years would literally be unconscious for four, five, or six hours. We didn't understand the physiology of the cardiovascular system or the respiratory system or the mechanics of blood flow, oxygenation, and fluid balance at all. People either got better or they didn't get better. But anesthesia's been a major force, it's walked side by side with the surgeon to protect his patients and allow them to recover.

"Then there've been the recovery rooms, the intensive care units. In the early days, the people who were critically ill—and could afford it—got the special-duty nurses. The special-duty nurses they turn out now have no concept of the management of all this technology they have in the units. Nursing down the line is going to be a big problem, because as hospitals get bigger, with more technology, you're going to have to turn to more paraprofessionals, people with technical expertise to take care of all this machinery," Mountain says.

Now, at day's end, when the hallways and all but two of the rooms are free of most human traffic, it is easy to see that the physical spaces of the Main O.R. are being overwhelmed by that proliferation of equipment and technology. Heavy-duty electrical extension cords crisscross many of the rooms like a living room during the holidays, proof that when these rooms were designed and built in the 1950s and 60s there was no need for all the outlets required by today's monitoring and powered surgical equipment. And rather than simply serve their intended purpose as indoor highways, the hallways of the Main O.R. have become equipment storage yards. Every evening, all the anesthesiologists' personal steel carts, which resemble the rolling chests used by garage mechanics, are lined up in one of the hallways, waiting for support staff to restock their drawers with the medications and supplies favored by each physician. Empty gurneys stand shoved against the walls, one used as a shelf to hold monitoring equipment that needs attention, another as a rolling linen closet.

"Right now the Main O.R. looks like a garage full of equipment," acknowledges hospital architect and interior designer Gerald Luss. In the midst of a major redesign, revamping, and expansion of the O.R. area, Luss notes: "The idea is to provide a very clearly defined environment, and hazard-free environment, for bringing the patient into the O.R. suite and treating the patient, and to make it as pleasing an area as possible esthetically, and part of doing that is the attention to the detail of the equipment and its storage and its accessibility when it's in use. It's one thing to walk into a room that just has an O.R. table in the middle of the room and the rest of the room is clean and clear, but if then when the patient is wheeled in all of a sudden all these other things have to come into it, you've defeated any advantage you have coming into a room that's wonderful architecturally.

"We're in the process right now of photographing and identifying every last piece of equipment that's in those corridors and sitting down with nursing and tracing what happens to that piece of equipment during a given period of time, where it goes," Luss explains. He says his solution to the storage problem entails creating "garages," spaces in the O.R. and hallway walls, for every piece of equipment that is now "homeless." "But if I garage something in one place," he says, "if that same piece of equipment is going to service this area and this, but also service a third place, they don't have the time to wheel it back to the first garage. So I have to provide garages on both sides of the O.R. area for the same piece of equipment. Because when they're through with it they're going to go to the nearest garage, or else they're going to leave it in the corridor. They have a very pragmatic problem—that's keeping the patient alive. That's all they worry about. They find the way it is now very self-defeating in terms of doing the job easily. They do the job very well, but it's not easy for them to do the job."

44

7:05 P.M. Lydia Slatalla's mechanical aortic valve will initially be held in place by ten stitches. Each suture Tony Tortolani has used is about twenty-four inches long and comes packaged with a tiny, curved cutting needle attached at each end. Gripping the needle with a needle holder, a scissorlike locking clamp about six inches long, Tortolani has worked his way around the aorta, alternately using blue and white sutures, running each of the sutures through a white cotton button, then through the wall of the aorta and back out through the wall and the button.

The aorta appears to form the center of a basket weaver's work-in-progress, with the weight of a series of clamps keeping tension on the now-doubled blue and white sutures tacked around that center. "Boy, she has a lot of calcium, Peter," Tortolani comments once again to anesthesiologist Walker. "She probably had rheumatic fever when she was a kid. Most people her age never knew they had rheumatic fever, they just had 'growing pains' for a month or so. Some got better, some didn't, but the damage from the fever is what triggers all this calcium buildup."

As Surgeon's Assistant Dom DiCapua suspends the mechanical valve above the aorta, using the valve holder packed with the device, Tortolani runs each of his sutures through the white Dacron cuff that runs around the rim of the valve. The alternating colors of the sutures allow him to keep the mess of thin lines in the right order. "Gently, men," Tortolani says, as he pulls the sutures tight and DiCapua lowers the valve into position.

At this moment the roller on the main pump of the heart-lung machine is turning at 2,800 revolutions per minute, sucking oxygen-depleted blood from Slatalla's body, passing it through the oxygenator and returning it to her system, at a rate of 4.2 liters per minute. Perfusionist Robin James is adding heparin to the system, on Tortolani's order, to slow clotting, because the current ACT, or active clotting time, is 412 seconds, and it should be about 480. So far, Lydia Slatalla has been given 10,000 units, a not unusual amount of the anti-clotting agent for such an operation.

Now Tortolani is tightening and tying off each of the sutures. The dissolving cotton button he has placed at each suture site protects the aortic wall and prevents him from tearing the delicate tissue as he works. "Robin, you want to give us some more cardioplegia, please," Tortolani orders. The temperature of the heart had gotten up to almost 63 degrees Fahrenheit, and Tortolani wants it brought back down to the 45 degree range. It is a truism that the safest amount of time for a patient to be on bypass is no time. While patients can be maintained by the machine for hours, many cardiac surgeons and researchers believe the use of the artificial device, which buffets the blood cells in its mechanical innards and circulates the blood in a steady flow, rather than in the pulsing manner of the heart, can have not-yet-understood, long-term, subtle neurological consequences. So it is important both to limit the time the pump is in use during surgery and to keep the patient's heart and circulatory system as cold as possible, to decrease the need for oxygenation and limit cell and tissue damage.

As Tortolani stands back, watching to see if his handiwork is holding properly, circulating nurse Karla Nash is making up charge slips for equipment and drugs that have been used on Lydia Slatalla to this point in the procedure. In its billing practices, the Main O.R. is not unlike a hot-sheets motel: for a flat half-hourly rate, the patient has the use of the room and a bed for whatever is going to be done; everything else is extra. As Nash records the items on charge slips similar to those used for standard credit cards, she imprints each slip with the patient's plastic hospital ID card. Slatalla has already been charged the hospital's cost, plus a 50 percent markup, for, among other things, a St. Jude's aortic valve, $5,512; a Hemovac suction pack, $126; a Swan Gans catheter and transducer, $112.50; a Cell Saver suction kit, $284.25; the disposable lines and filters used thus far for the heart-lung machine, $873; foam elbow pads, $18; two O.R. packs—which include the drapes and towels covering the operating table and instrument stands—$87; two grams of Kefzol, an antibiotic, $5.79; two grams of Kantrex, another antibiotic, $54.57; 50 milli-grams of Nipride, to increase cardiac output, $2.60; 50 milligrams of Tridil, a form of nitroglycerine, for a mere $.71; and 20 milligrams of Levophed, to help regulate blood pressure, at $55.05. And that $7,129.47 does not include the bills for the room itself, the surgeon, the anes-thesiologist, the surgeon's assistant, the blood, packed cells, saline, or any of the sutures, sponges, or other supplies that have been, and will be, used during the operation.

This is going to be quite a shopping spree.

45

7:54 P.M. The five slightly dirty toes of Louis Morales's left foot poking forlornly from beneath the blue-and-green surgical drapes at one end of the operating table, and a saucer-shaped disc of the bloody tissue that would normally be hidden by his dark brown hair and scalp, rising like a red moon from the sea of drapes at the opposite end, are the only hints of the urgent business under way in Room 12. That and a series of twenty-four CAT scan images of the teenager's skull attached to the viewing box on one of the room's tile walls. It doesn't take a neurosurgeon to recognize two of the black spots on the CAT scans as bullet fragments lodged in Morales's brain. It will, however, take a neurosurgeon to remove them.

A series of four Yaserville scalp hooks, anchored with a series of springs and wires to the instrument table suspended above the teenager's chest, hold back part of the scalp; surgical clamps anchor the rest. "It's an orbital entrance wound, and there's spinal fluid coming out of it," neurosurgeon David Chalif tells Larry Walsh, one of the surgeon's assistants who work for Long Island Neurosurgery Associates.

After drilling a burr hole just above and in front of the

right ear, Chalif uses a small power saw in the burr hole and cuts a circular trap door, about the size of an orange, in the top of the skull. "Everything okay over there?" he asks anesthesiologist Robert LaPorta.

"Sleeping like a baby. Which he is," comes the reply. LaPorta is the anesthesiologist on-call tonight, which means he reported for work at 5:00 P.M. and will go home when relieved by the day shift at seven tomorrow morning. LaPorta and the on-call anesthesiologist up in the labor and delivery suite can provide backup for each other or, if it proves to be a wild night, call in help. This emergency admission, so early in the evening, is not a good sign, LaPorta thinks.

David Chalif lifts the top off Louis Morales's skull and uses forceps and a small suction tube to lift lead fragments off the dura, the protective covering of the brain. According to the police report, the youngster said he was accidentally shot with a BB gun, but these silvery-gray lead fragments, and the size of the hole in his skull, weren't left by a BB. "Here's the entrance wound," Chalif announced, "and here's the hole in the dura where the bullet went in."

46

On the side of Robert LaPorta's anesthesia cart there is a piece of plastic label tape that reads, ROB LAPORTA IS A NICE GUY. While that is the general assessment of LaPorta by those who work in the Main O.R., the odds are overwhelming that the message, which the anesthesiologist clearly appreciates, was placed there by a nurse.

"Don't ever let anybody kid you," LaPorta says. "Nurses run the O.R. Nurses run the hospital. Nurses can cause the O.R. to speed up; or, they can make it slow down. Don't believe anything else. 'We can't start the case now, it's lunch break.' Nobody says to me, 'Have you had your lunch yet, Dr. LaPorta?' If they want to burn you, they can burn you. 'The room isn't cleaned yet.' They don't clean the room, but they get it done. 'We can't find the equipment.' If they want it, they find it. They can speed it up the same way. They get the room turned around faster, get everything ready. I get along with the nurses, but I have my run-ins. If I think something isn't safe, I won't do it. A lot of the surgeons come in with this 'I'm the surgeon here' attitude. Or 'I'm the anesthesiologist.' People then go out of their way to make it difficult for those people.

"Beginning with my internship at Nassau County Medical Center, I learned early on, don't burn anybody," LaPorta recalls. "There were some guys who would come in and say, 'I'm the doctor,' and that was it for the rest of the year there—they were dead meat. The nurses would call them for anything: 'I thought you'd like to know that Mrs. Soandso's asleep now!' I never got those calls, and sometimes the nurses were helpful to me."

It was predictable that LaPorta, with a master's in electronmicroscopy and a Ph.D. in oral biology/pathology, would shine at Nassau County Medical Center [NCMC], Long Island's only county hospital. What was not at all predictable was that he would have those credentials.

LaPorta's background is so jarringly at odds with his academic and professional accomplishments that he refers to himself only half-jokingly as the "white sheep in the family." The son of a truck mechanic, Rob LaPorta is one of only two of six children in the family to graduate from high school, and is the only one who graduated from college. A fat child who found solace and companionship in books, to this day he remembers an initial trip to the main library in Freeport, where he grew up on Long Island.

"I'd always gone to the bookmobile, but when we took that trip to the library I still remember the thrill of realizing there were so many books. It was a very magical moment. I just couldn't believe there were so many books in the world," he recalls.

"I was never really pushed to go to college or anything. I just wanted to go. So I made all the decisions, applied to all the schools, saved money. Undergraduate was strange. I was very interested in physics and astronomy, so I spent about six months at the University of Arizona. But I quickly realized two things: I couldn't handle the math, and I was rapidly running out of money. So a friend of mine said, 'Why don't you go to Hofstra, where I'm going, and study biology? There's very little math involved.' So I went to Hofstra second semester, lived at home and worked in the Freeport library, just the way I did in high school, to pay

my way through college. It took me five years to get
through school because I could only afford to go part-time.
It was kind of fun, but it wasn't your typical college thing.
I would go to classes, and whenever I didn't have class I'd
work. I also did odd jobs to get money. I did everything
at the library: I drove the bookmobile, I put the books away
on the shelves, Saturday morning I waxed the floor, I took
care of the film collection—you name it, I did it. And it
was a great place, because for somebody who's interested
in books, where else would you be?

"So I majored in biology," LaPorta says, noting that his
interest in astronomy continues to this day, fueled by a
home telescope and dark backyard. "I was trying to figure
out what to do. It was in the middle of the draft thing, but
my number was 356. A girl in college told me about a free
year-long program at NCMC where you ended up with a
degree in medical technology. So I did that for a year
during the day and worked in the library at night. Then I
got a job working midnight to eight in the NCMC Emergency Room lab. And that's where I met Doretta," whom
he married. "We were on the same shift and we were the
only ones there. Anyway, while I was working there I was
working on my master's degree in electronmicroscopy at
Hofstra. I've always been mechanically inclined, so that
worked out real well. In two years I got a master's, and for
the last year they farm you out, and they sent me to Cold
Spring Harbor Laboratory. I did some research there, finished my master's there, and then worked at Cold Spring
Harbor for six months while I applied for my Ph.D. program."

LaPorta ended up in a doctoral program at the State
University of New York at Stony Brook and spent half his
time there and half his time at Cold Spring Harbor, where,
because he used the facility's word processing program to
write his thesis as he moved along through the Ph.D. program, he earned the degree in three years, rather than the
usual four to six, and published a number of papers along

the way. "All my postdoc friends at Cold Spring Harbor were having a hard time finding jobs—this was like '79 to '82," he says. "Everybody was saying they couldn't find a job, and one guy found a job at the University of Mississippi and said he might have tenure in a couple of years. I said, 'This is not a good idea.' I was married by then and I said to Doretta, 'Maybe I'll apply to medical school, it's got to be a steady job, we'll never starve.' I decided to take the MCATs [Medical College Admission Test], which is a story in itself because I hadn't taken organic chemistry in seven years." But LaPorta just went back to the library and then aced his MCATs. He was accepted at George Washington University Medical School, but the tuition was $19,000. So he was back at the State University at Stony Brook, where the medical school tuition was $4,000 a year and he taught in the Biology Department for his first two years.

Through the "wonders of the match system," LaPorta ended up doing a year's internship in medicine back at NCMC, and then he was off to Boston and the heady world of Harvard and Brigham and Women's Hospital. "No one at Stony Brook had pushed us toward anesthesia," he says. "There were only four out of one hundred of us who wanted to go into it. But I just liked anesthesia. I was probably in an O.R. once and had seen all this machinery and I love machinery. I'm not the kind of person who wants to solve these little picayune problems. Internal medicine people have these lists of differential diagnoses, and it's very slow. You give somebody medicine and wait a few days to see if something happens. People get slightly better or they don't. You maybe switch medicines. It was kind of boring. And I didn't like dealing with the patients all the time. You feel kind of helpless. You're not really helping them that much, or that fast. And surgery? I couldn't really deal with the ego structure I found in a lot of surgeons. I think what turned me off was that during medical school I spent my surgical rotation at NCMC, and they weren't very good, they weren't very happy people, and they

treated us like total shit. Most of the time you weren't in
the O.R., you were upstairs drawing blood and stuff. One
summer I arranged to do a special rotation in anesthesia
at Stony Brook for a month, and I really liked it. I said,
'Hey, you're really good. You know what you're doing.' So
that's why I went into anesthesia. I also liked the fact you
saw the patient the night before, you had the operation,
and you saw them the day after, and asked, 'How are you
doing?' So it was cut and dry. It had a beginning point and
an end point. The patients didn't come back again because
they still had their high blood pressure or their gout was
bothering them for the eighth month in a row. I guess I'm
the kind of person that doesn't like dealing with patients
that much except in a one-time situation. I don't want them
to come back to me complaining."

For the kid from Freeport, a residency at Brigham and
Women's was like a job in a candy factory. "I had the most
wonderful residency I could ever have asked for," LaPorta
says. "We worked very hard, we certainly complained, but
they really knew how to take care of you there. The chairman, Dr. Benjamin Covino, who died recently, was one of
the wonderful men in the world. It was like your dad was
there—if you happen to like your dad. The minute you
walked in, he knew who you were. In a short while, he
knew your wife's name, he knew your kids' names. He went
out of his way to ask how you were doing. He used to be
away a lot, but whenever he was there he was in the O.R.,
directing the floor. Most chairmen of academic departments are never in the O.R., but he was always there whenever he was in Boston. The biggest fear I had going to
Brigham was it was going to be a really snobby place. My
background didn't include places like that. I figured it
would be 'Look at this funny Long Island Italian kid.' But
they were very nice. They really made you feel like family.
It was a wonderful, wonderful experience, but all those
experiences end. I was really tempted to stay there. I went
in to ask Dr. Covino for a letter of recommendation, and

he said, 'We'd love to have you here.' I knew they'd love to have me there, but the money I'd make there would pale by comparison to what I'd make anywhere else." As a clinical instructor in anesthesia at Harvard, LaPorta says, he would have been making about $90,000 a year, and after five or six years would be making about $110,000, a salary half or a third of what it would be in a private group. So after completing his three-year residency in anesthesia and fellowship in obstetrical anesthesia in only two and a half years, because he got credit for having a Ph.D., he moved back to Long Island and North Shore.

"You come in as an employee for four years and the salary goes up very slowly, and then you become a partner. I started in January of 1990. A lot of these guys have incredible amounts of money. They were working in a time when you could sock away as much money as you wanted in the pension plan, so they put away incredible amounts of money. They bought their house for $60,000. You won't see that kind of money in the future anymore. It bothers me, but that's okay. As an employee of the group I'm making around $135,000. The average is several times that, but with the changes coming in the way we pay for medical care, I'll never go that high, which is fine," LaPorta says, noting that he doesn't even know what he earns for a given case. "I just put down when a case starts and when it ends. The way it works is the difficulty of the case determines a flat rate, and then it's how many hours it lasts, divided into fifteen-minute blocks. There's a base rate for the type of surgery, plus the fifteen-minute blocks. The amount charged per fifteen-minute block is the same for all types of surgery. It's a lot of money. It's probably more than most physicians make, except for the surgeons. But a lot of guys in medicine can't make it on $400,000. They have ex-wives, three mortgages, and if the income goes down by $150,000 they'll be in deep shit. But Doretta and I don't have expensive dreams. I think poor. My father didn't have a very good job. We were always living on the edge. We were taught never to waste money. Doretta and I fight constantly about my being too cheap. Our car can last another year, there's nothing wrong with it. Which is probably why I went into medicine, because I was afraid. I was fighting for security. It was the most secure job I could think of. I don't live ostentatiously. This last year and a half, what we've been doing is bringing all our debts down. Paying off medical school loans. Paying off our credit cards. Paying our mortgage faster than we have to."

While LaPorta is willing to acknowledge the kind of salaries that physicians, particularly in his specialty, earn, he has no apologies to make for that pay scale. "Yes, I can work one twenty-four-hour shift taking call for the partners in the group and get paid as much as I get paid for working two weeks. But do we get paid too much? I don't think so. Are baseball players paid too much? They don't think so. I certainly am not going to turn down somebody paying me more money. But Doretta will tell you that when we bought this house, for a good six months I said we shouldn't really live here, it's not our place. I still do feel that in a way. I'm very hesitant to show people I own this"—his modern five-bedroom house. "Maybe I'm blowing up this house in my mind," he wonders. "Certainly physicians have bigger houses. I'm sure it's my upbringing. But the guy next to me is in business. Does he deserve that much money? I know that people who are less qualified now are going into medicine because they see the rewards. I went into it for security. Does security equal income? Yes. I'll always have an income. I could get a job when and wherever. We may have a smaller house, but we'll always eat. Especially in anesthesia. I could leave and join another group."

Despite having done his fellowship in obstetrical anesthesia, LaPorta, one of Peter Walker's "young Turks," resists concentrating in that area at North Shore because he says that if he did, he would very quickly lose his skills in other areas, something he is loath to do. But he does get great satisfaction from working in the labor and delivery area. "Very few of us do OB anesthesia, because it's a different kind of anesthesia. You're dealing with unpremedicated, screaming women who are in a lot of pain. You can't give them a lot of medicine. You can't give them Valium. And you have to get this epidural into a moving target. Once you do that it's okay. But then you have to deal with the baby. You have to know neonatal resuscitation, and that can be hairy. A lot of people won't go up to OB. When the group was formed out of what was basically a collection of freelancers, different people had specialties. Peter did hearts. Dominic would always do neuro. Glen would do OB. Nalan would do pediatrics. But when the group came together, they tried to mix them around. Mike Myers says the important thing isn't the operation, it's the medical condition of the patient, and he's right. Are you doing a knee repair on a nineteen-year-old athlete, or a seventy-three-year-old with severe cardiovascular disease. The knee may be the same, but the patient sure isn't.

"Take people with vascular diseases who need surgery," LaPorta continues. "They didn't get those vascular diseases from clean living. If their arteries in their legs are in rotten shape, you can be sure the arteries in their heart are in rotten shape. So those are the hairy operations. A gallbladder? It could be a healthy patient, but it could also be a very sick patient. We're the internists of the O.R. Patients who come into the O.R., especially from an I.C.U. or something, leave in better medical shape than when they came in. They're more tuned up. The fluid balances are better. Even in an I.C.U. setting you don't have one doctor working on one patient continuously. The I.C.U. patients are just non-asleep surgical patients. A lot of them are on ventilators, which anesthesia understands very well. A lot of them are on a lot of different drips, dopamine and whatnot. A lot of them have medical problems that the surgeons don't appreciate. We don't have as much ego as a surgeon does," he says. "We're comfortable sitting down behind our curtain. 'You do the work, that's fine. We'll take care of the patient.'

"Trauma is stressful, but it may be one of the least stressful forms of anesthesia. I hate to say it, but if the patient dies, it's not the world's worst thing. It's terrible for the patient, but it's not necessarily your fault. You do a gallbladder and somebody dies on the table, somebody screwed up big time. You do a guy who's shot five times and he dies, 'I'm sorry, we tried our best.' It is exciting. I like it, but I wouldn't quite call it fun. It's more like you're using your skills, there's an edge. Inside you say, 'I'm good.' When you do a gallbladder, and everything goes well, you're good, but so's the guy next to you. But when you get a guy through a difficult trauma, you can say, 'That was good.' Trauma's also easy in a way, because what you're doing is giving them lots of fluid, keeping up with blood loss, keeping the heart and kidneys going. It's rote. You're not worried about getting them through with perfect electrolytes, you're worried about getting them out alive. Also, most trauma patients are young, and they're tremendously resilient.

"In fact," LaPorta says, "sometimes in major trauma you don't give anesthesia, you just give oxygen and paralyze them. I know it sounds horrible, but they don't remember what happened. If you're not giving them anesthesia, it's because their blood pressure's so low that you can't depress it any more. And when it's that low, it may be that the brain isn't getting as much oxygen" [as it needs for perception of pain]. As the blood pressure rises, he says, the anesthesiologist begins adding drugs to block pain, which can also depress the respiratory and cardiovascular systems. "But doing anesthesia is not like some magical thing. It's just human beings doing it. After a while it becomes very routine. It's like the first rocket to the moon. The first time it's 'Wow, isn't that incredible!' But after a while it becomes routine. On the other hand, we can't have a down day. If you have a down day you have to be there. You have to be one hundred percent, and people are only human. It eats away at you. Everybody says, talking to doctors, 'What pressure do you have? It's not your ass in the operating room. You're not on that table. Where's the pressure?' No, you don't die. But you sure don't want to screw up. It's also an ego thing too: 'I can't screw up, I'm the doctor.' Most people in medicine are very intelligent, very egotistical. They don't want to think they could ever fail.

"I don't think you should ever feel really comfortable," LaPorta contends. "I feel stress for my patients. Little kids bother me a lot because I have my own two children. The thought of something happening to a little kid is just horrible. But I worry about all my patients. Do I ever think that this could be the one that doesn't wake up? All the time. I don't know if everybody does, but I worry about it all the time. But the thing with anesthesia is you try to get yourself prepared for what can happen. 'This patient has asthma, what can happen that is gonna go wrong and how can I, first, prevent it from happening and, second, treat it if it occurs?' Like, I give all my patients a drug to help keep their stomach empty, to keep them from getting nauseous and aspirating, which can be a terminal event. They all get that. Has that decreased the chances of aspiration? Maybe, and hopefully it's for the good.

"I try to be very conscientious about what I do," LaPorta says. "I try not to cut corners too much, although there's time pressure and you cut corners. You can always write down more than you do, you can always document better than you document, but then you would spend hours writing things and you couldn't get anything done. I try to keep it contemporaneous because I'm compulsive about that. But it is a game, it's who's going to believe whom. That's probably one of the reasons why I hate lawyers. I'm reviewing four different anesthesia cases now where people are being sued for malpractice. In most of the cases it appears to me that there wasn't anything done that, if somebody else had done it, wouldn't have gone wrong exactly the same way. I hate to say it, but I think of it as a game, and whoever puts up the best front is the guy who wins. What I'm saying is the legal process is not what it says it is: it's not there to define the truth and give justice. For anybody to think anything else is bullshit. They're so duplicitous. When they work for you it's great, when they don't, they're bastards. They're not there to find the truth and get justice. They're there to win, no matter how they do it, no matter how they can cheat. It's not justice. It's a game. If you go to a lot of doctors and ask, 'Are you going to let your kids go into medicine?' they say, 'Not if I can help it.' And it's because of malpractice."

While the malpractice situation has made the life of the anesthesiologist more difficult over the past decade, technology has brought it vast improvements. "A lot of the technology we use has really gotten good," LaPorta says. "And the pharmacology has improved, the number of drugs we use, even the muscle relaxants. A lot of the old muscle relaxants caused tachycardia or bradycardia [increased and decreased heart rate], which you don't want. The beta-blockers help preserve blood pressure and heart rate, and now we have a garbage list of them. The technology's improved. Instantaneous blood pressure monitoring has improved. We have lines to monitor ischemia. Pulse oxymeters are new, that's one of God's greatest gifts to anesthesia." A tiny spring-loaded device that slips over one of the patient's fingertips, the pulse oxymeter uses a pulse of light to measure the blood oxygen saturation, a vast improvement over the anesthesiologist's observing the color of the fingernails while waiting for the lab to send back the results of a blood-gas analysis. "On the other hand," LaPorta adds, "with all the advances we've made, to this day nobody really understands how the gases work. There are different theories, but each of the theories has different flaws that show that the theories aren't one hundred percent correct.

"It's funny," Rob LaPorta says, "but a lot of people still

think that we roll them into a room, put some stuff in their veins and leave. I'm very serious. I think they think we're not there anymore. But putting them to sleep is the easy part. Kids and adults are both scared of anesthesia, but for opposite reasons: kids are frightened of anesthesia because they're afraid they're going to wake up before the operation is done. They're afraid of feeling pain or being awake when somebody's doing something. It's just the opposite with adults. With adults, it's the fear that they won't wake up. I'm afraid of it. I would avoid anesthesia at all costs. I have this terrible nose condition, deviated septum and nasal polyps. I haven't breathed through my nose in years. I've looked, I'm an acceptable anesthesia risk, I'd be an easy intubation, but I'm scared. Part of that can be the old physician control thing—physicians always have to be in control. Also, I have a morbid personality, and sometimes I wonder if people are awake, but just don't show it, and then forget everything after the operation. We have EEGs and things that show that the state of the brain is different, but your body is aware. When you cut into it, your blood pressure goes up. And I avoid high-risk things. But, as I say to all my patients, there's more risk in driving to work than there is having anesthesia."

47

8:15 P.M. Lydia Slatalla's heart is once again pumping blood through her circulatory system, much more efficiently now that the mechanical valve has replaced her calcified aortic valve, although the lines for the heart-lung machine are still in place—just in case. Two half-inch diameter, Silastic drainage tubes have each been shoved through incisions in the chest wall on either side of her body, and Tony Tortolani is now using the Bouvie cautery to seal off bleeders along the edge of the pericardium, the protective sac around the heart.

The surgeon and the anesthesiologist are talking about the changing sociopolitical world of medicine, and Peter Walker has been telling Tortolani about his son's experiences as a premed student. "He's a wonderfully gregarious kid, who's good with people," Walker says. "He's now discovering how much work it is, and he hasn't bailed out yet."

"How do you feel about him doing it, Peter?"

"I'm on the fence," Walker says.

"Come off bypass," Tortolani tells perfusionist Robin James.

"I'm off."

"Transfuse."

"Transfusing," she tells him, pumping back to Lydia Slatalla the last unit of her blood that was scavenged during surgery by the Cell Saver attached to the heart-lung machine.

Tortolani inserts a probe, connected to one of the monitors, into Slatalla's aorta. "One-twenty-nine over sixty-three," he announces, clearly pleased.

"Just goes to prove my theory," Walker says "You've got to have three things in this business: you've got to have a good surgeon, good rhythm—and a good ventricle."

Vinnie Parnell, who was seeing patients late in the afternoon and then stayed to clean up paperwork, sticks his head around the door of Room 3, holding a mask in place over his nose and mouth. "How's she doing?" he asks his partner.

"Okay now, but it was a struggle," Tortolani answers. "It took me about twenty minutes to cut away enough calcium to wedge in a nineteen St. Jude's."

"But you got it in?"

"Finally."

"All right. I'll see you in the morning. You operating early?"

"Not tomorrow. I've got meetings starting at seven."

"Okay, I'll talk to you sometime around noon, if you've got a minute. Take it easy. Good night, all."

"Night, Vinnie."

48

8:40 P.M. "The bullet either went through or under the falx," David Chalif says, gently probing the surface of Louis Morales's brain. Chalif has already sliced through the dura and sewn it to small holes he has created around the edges of the opening he cut in the skull. "Becky, don't lose this —it's a bullet fragment," the neurosurgeon says, dropping the ragged bit of metal onto a white surgical sponge offered by scrub nurse Rebecca Richmond.

"I'm creating an area of resection here," Chalif tells anesthesiologist Rob LaPorta, who can't see what Chalif is doing because of the position of the operating field. "It's not very elegant brain surgery, but it's all we can do at this point. This tissue is destroyed beyond repair. Well, the bullet crossed the midline below the falx," he says. "See, Larry, here's the falx," the portion of the dura that runs between the right and left hemispheres. He points to the path the bullet has cut though the grayish-white brain tissue, and continues to remove bits of damaged, and contaminated, tissue from the frontal lobe, the area of the brain that is the seat of personality and conscious thought. "Wow! The bullet went right over the anterior cerebral artery!" Chalif announces. "We're definitely going to need an angiogram down the road here. I'm not worried about this little stuff, I'm worried about the major arteries."

It is now 9:00 P.M., and circulating nurse Nadine Cristo has swung the Zeiss operating microscope into position above the opening in Louis Morales's skull. "We're ready for Jim Firstman," Chalif says. "I think he's in the O.R. at Long Island Jewish." Cristo calls the front desk on the Room 12 phone and asks that the plastic and reconstructive surgeon, who was alerted earlier, be told that he's needed.

"Is he going to have trouble playing chess?" surgical resident Peter Marks asks, facetiously.

But he's surprised when Calif says, "No, believe it or not, I don't think he'll have any serious problems, depending on what else was damaged."

Jim Firstman, who was in his car between the two hospitals when he was called, walks into the room. Chalif offers Firstman a stool, and the plastic surgeon peers into Louis Morales's brain. The bullet hole looms large on the upper left edge of the opening of the skull, a red-rimmed, white circle. Below it, the brain is a tangle of pink and white, with bright red patches. The most prominent features Firstman can see through the optics are two arteries, and the path of the bullet literally just beneath the arteries. If either had been nicked, or is nicked in the O.R. . . .

"That whole frontal area should be stripped off," Firstman tells Chalif.

"What's the chance that bullet won't cause him any problem?" Peter Marks asks.

"The path shouldn't," Chalif says, "and the bullet shouldn't. It could be a site of infection, but I'm more worried about swelling." And more worried still about the damage that could be caused by any attempt to remove the fragment. "He may lose his sense of smell, and his taste could be affected, too, but we'll just have to wait and see. But the fact that he was awake when he came in here was a good sign."

It takes Chalif less than twenty minutes to remove the

damaged tissue and begin to close the dura. "How do you want to fill that hole?" Firstman asks the neurosurgeon, referring to the bullet hole in the dura.

"Just leave it as a hole."

"I'd be inclined to close that hole, David, because he'll be left with a divot."

As Chalif works on the dura, Firstman tells Chalif, "We have to have a very long talk, David. Very long and very private."

"About Sarah?"

"Yes, about Sarah."

"When do you think you'll be out of here?" one of the night nurses calls from the doorway to Room 12, ending the cryptic exchange.

"Another hour and a half," Chalif tells her.

"I saw you this morning, Jim," Chalif says, glancing up for a moment. "What were you doing?"

"I was getting ready to reconstruct a vagina. But she turned out to have positive lymph nodes, so we couldn't do it. We had to do a total pelvic exenteration," which is the removal of all the organs in the pelvis.

"God. How old was she?"

"She's forty-seven years old, has six kids. And she's a nice woman."

It is 9:52. The dura is closed and has been flushed with saline solution, and Jim Firstman takes over. He is now the only surgeon working in the sixteen rooms of the Main O.R. Work ended in Room 3 about twenty minutes ago. Tony Tortolani has gone home, and Peter Walker will leave shortly. Firstman snips out the back wall of the sinus the bullet passed through, and he now begins cleaning out the mucosa.

Fifty minutes later, it's David Chalif's case again. It takes him about an hour and a half, until about 11:30, to close up the wounds he created treating the wounds the bullet caused. He has to wire into place the piece of skull he removed, and then stitch the scalp back into place. If it is not technically demanding work, it is slow, tedious going. As he finishes, Chalif dramatically yanks back a portion of the drapes covering the patient and there lies a child. The faint beginnings of a mustache darken the white skin of his upper lip, and incredibly long thick lashes fall below his closed eyes. A tiny red spot above his right eyebrow, barely more than a pimple, marks the entrance wound.

Now Chalif is trying to arrange for another CAT scan but is having problems. He has been told the front desk is calling the radiology resident. "What are you calling the resident for? The resident has to approve it? That's bullshit! You call the resident and tell him it's a stat scan," he tells Nadine Cristo. "And if someone says we can't get a scan because the computer is down, the person who says the computer is down is going to need a scan!"

49

11:56 P.M. First-year surgical resident Arnie Newman sits at the nursing station, an island of light in the darkened Post Anesthesia Care Unit—the Recovery Room. Only three of the seventeen beds in the unit are occupied at this late hour, and John Guthrie, the alcoholic, eighty-two-year-old patient in one of the three, is the focus of Newman's attention.

The white-coated resident is slumped forward over the counter, his left hand simultaneously cradling a telephone receiver and propping up his head. "This is Arnie. Sorry to bother you," he tells the senior resident, who over the years of nights on-call has been awakened so often to hear that phrase that he has come to wonder if "Sorrytobotheryou" might not be his first name. "You know John?" Newman asks his sleepy chief at the other end of the line. "Right. Well, he's awake, alert and moving. But . . . well, he won't talk. No, nothing. We don't know whether he's bullshitting us, or he's aphasic"—unable to speak due to a cerebrovascular "accident," usually a stroke. This afternoon Guthrie successfully underwent surgery to remove a blockage in his left carotid artery, which is one of the two primary blood supplies to the brain.

In response to a question asked by his chief, Arnie Newman glances over his shoulder toward Guthrie. "He's clapping his hands now," he says. And indeed Guthrie is. The gaunt old man, who with his hawklike visage and shock of pure white hair could pass for John Brown in an old daguerreotype, is up on one elbow, angrily clapping his hands at the two nurses at his bedside, apparently attempting to chase them away. "Well, he's quite cooperative. You want to talk to him? I don't know, I can hand him the phone and trick him into it." He laughs at the thought. "No, it won't reach over there." Newman puts the phone down, pushes himself up and shuffles over to Guthrie's bed. "John? Dr. Reich is on the phone. Do you want to talk to him?" The old man shakes his head emphatically from side to side.

Newman walks back to the desk and picks up the receiver again. "Peter? He said he doesn't know you. He shook his head no." He listens for a few moments and then says, "There's only two things we can do. We can give him some heparin [to thin his blood] or we can take him back to the O.R." Newman listens again and then relays a question to the nurses. "Will he stick his tongue out?" he calls over to the bedside.

"He would before," assistant head nurse Jackie Sirica tells Newman. "He'd move and stick his tongue out, but not since he's stopped talking."

"Okay," Newman says, and he hangs up the phone and walks back over to Guthrie's bed. The young resident attempts to place his hands on the patient's abdomen, but John Guthrie shakes his head, draws away, and angrily shakes his fist. "Come on, John," Newman says in that loud voice the young reserve for the old, who they assume are all either deaf or stupid. "I'm not going to hurt you. I just want to examine you." But the old man is having none of it.

Now Arnie Newman, who wants desperately to escape to the on-call room and sleep, is on the phone to the neurology resident on-call. "Yes, he obeys commands and he communicates with motions. I'm wondering, is it possible to have complete speech deficit without any other symptoms?"

Guthrie continues to gesture, repeatedly making a child's hand signal for "crazy" and pointing at himself. Whenever Newman looks toward Guthrie, the patient places a thumb in each ear and wiggles his hands in a gesture of derision. Jackie Sirica attempts to remove a stray piece of tape from Guthrie's forehead, but each time she reaches forward, he jerks back, becoming extremely agitated. Then, every time she turns away from the bed, he calms down and pulls his covers up to his chin. If all of this is simply a lonely old man's way of getting attention, it is succeeding. This little drama has gone on for more than an hour, and Dr. Sanjay Pasha, senior neurology resident, has just walked into the unit.

After briefing Pasha, Newman slumps back down at the nursing station and, with his head in his hands, mutters, "I can't believe I'm staying awake to deal with this."

50

1:03 A.M. There have certainly been worse nights than this, Rob LaPorta thinks. There was, after all, the night the Avianca jet slammed into the hillside in nearby Cove Neck, turning the Main O.R. into a scene from Dante's *Inferno*. On the other hand, if a good night on-call is a rented movie on the VCR in the Anesthesia Department office and eight hours sleep on the lumpy foldout couch, then this is not a good night.

Here it is, after 1:00 A.M., and LaPorta hasn't had a break, other than to go to the bathroom or to grab a cup of day-old coffee, since coming on duty eight hours ago, and now he is preparing for another procedure, laying out his drugs on the tabletop that is part of the Narkomed 2B anesthesia machine in Room 10. He has already drawn the medications and has laid the filled and labeled syringes out in groups.

For emergencies, there is atropine to speed up the heart, lidocaine to control irregular heart rhythms, ephedrine and Neo-Synephrine to increase the blood pressure, and Normodyne to lower the blood pressure; for pain, the narcotic Fentanyl; to insure amnesia, the powerful, Valium-like tranquilizer midazolam; to relax the muscles and induce paralysis, Pavulon, Vercuronium, and two syringes of Anectine; and, for sleep, penathol.

LaPorta has already turned on the anesthesia machine, checked its circuits, and adjusted the volume on the ventilator, setting it higher than he normally would so that it will move a larger than usual amount of oxygen-laden air to the patient's lungs, "because he's a bigger guy," says LaPorta, who, at six feet and over two hundred pounds, is a big guy himself.

The patient, Richard Arnold, is a 220-pound, six foot, forty-five-year-old who fell off a ladder in his home earlier in the evening. Like many accident victims, he postponed coming to the hospital, thinking that whatever he had done to himself would "get better." But the badly fractured humerus in his left arm didn't miraculously set itself, so now he is lying on a gurney in the hallway outside Room 10. "Mr. Arnold? I'm Dr. LaPorta, from Anesthesia. I'm going to ask you a bunch of questions everybody's probably asked you, okay? Are you allergic to any drugs?"

"No," Arnold mumbles.

"Good. Now, I'm going to read a list of things, and if any of them apply to you, say so." LaPorta then reads the standard list of medical conditions and complications— Arnold says no to all of them—and LaPorta tells the patient: "I'm going to give you a drug to make you drowsy. Then we'll talk." He injects Versed, a powerful tranquilizer and amnesia-inducing drug, into the IV line that was placed in Arnold's wrist in the Emergency Room. He also gives Arnold the drug Reglan, which will reduce nausea. Next come the warnings.

"It's possible to damage teeth when we put in the tube, but I've never done it," LaPorta tells his patient. "There's always the chance of something catastrophic happening, death, stroke," brain damage or damage to any number of other vital organs. In fact, LaPorta has never had an anesthesia accident and has never experienced the death of a patient on the table. While there is no question that, nationally, a surgery patient is far more likely to be killed by an anesthesia accident than by a surgical "misadventure," and while the risk of anesthesia death during surgery is put at one in ten thousand, anesthesia death in the Main O.R. is so rare as to be statistically all but impossible.

It is 1:30. Orthopedic surgeon Irvin Spira, who arrived at the hospital a few minutes ago, is checking the equipment laid out by the two nurses working the case, Jack Reynolds, who will scrub, and Kevin McCarthy, who's circulating: a battery-driven drill and four battery packs; three chucks for the drill, including an angle driver; titanium rods for insertion in Arnold's arm; Styker reamers—specialty drill bits. Having examined X rays taken earlier, Spira has decided to repair Arnold's arm with intramedulary, or I.M., rodding. Where joining the two ends of the bone together with metal plates and screws would involve a large incision, this operation, which involves drilling a vertical tunnel through the humerus and inserting a rod, will call for an opening of only about an inch and a half in the top of the arm. "The fracture's near the end of the bone. It *should* heal well. On the other hand, this type of fracture is known for nonunion," the surgeon says.

After placing a large, black O.R. equivalent of a beanbag on the table, for help in positioning the patient, Spira and LaPorta slide Arnold from his gurney to the operating table. Despite their care and the narcotics he has been given, the patient grunts with pain as his arm is moved.

An hour and twenty minutes after LaPorta began setting up, Richard Arnold is asleep on the operating table, in a sitting, "beach chair" position. The "beanbag," which was placed between his back and the table, was temporarily hooked to the room's suction line, allowing the staff to create a vacuum in the bag and mold it to Arnold's back and sides, to help hold him steady in the sitting position. His right arm is extended to the side, supported by an extension of the table. And the table itself has been turned from its normal position in the room, so that it now faces two viewing monitors that are used with the Philips BV 25 portable C-arm fluoroscope, which will be used during surgery to allow the surgeons to follow the rod as they drive it through the humerus. As LaPorta watches Spira literally staple the drapes to the flesh around the top of Arnold's arm, the anesthesiologist admits; "My personal preference would be to have a spinal or epidural—anything to be awake—because I don't want to trust my life to someone else."

Spira, who, like everyone else in the room is wearing a lead-lined vest and collar for protection from the fluoroscope's radiation, makes his initial incision with the electric cautery. That done, he begins the carpentry, first boring into the head of the humerus with an enormous steel awl. Once he is through the bone, orthopedic resident Bill Potter taps a guide wire through the hollow center of the two pieces of the fractured humerus, using the flouroscopic pictures as a guide.

"Can I have the tissue protector and the number four reamer?" Spira says to the scrub nurse, who hands him the power drill with a long, flexible rod, ending in a bone-cutting bit, locked in the chuck. Working a short distance at a time, Spira uses the reamer to enlarge the channel down the center of the bone and continually pulls the bit out and slides a guide wire, the diameter of the rod he will be using, into the channel.

It is 3:03 A.M. Bill Potter is using a steel mallet with plastic end caps to hammer a titanium rod—stronger and lighter than steel—into place in Richard Arnold's arm. As the fluoroscope shows the rod approaching the point of the break, Spira manipulates the two pieces so that Potter can drive the rod home, through the break and into the lower portion of the bone. It takes just twelve minutes to complete the job. As Spira is stitching up the small incision at the top of the patient's arm, LaPorta is adding Kefzol, a member of the cephalosporin family of antibiotics. "Sometimes, at the end of a case, they tell me to give whatever the cephalosporin du jour is," LaPorta says. Arnold, who will not have to wear a cast, will remain in the hospital for about two days, on IV antibiotics, and then will be sent home. In a week he'll go to Spira's office to have the stitches removed.

"Richard! Richard! Come on, Richard, wake up," LaPorta calls to the patient. "Come on, Richard. Time to get up." He adds some Narcan to the IV to reverse some, but not all, of the effect of the narcotics he had administered. The patient bucks, fighting the endotracheal tube in his throat, but does not open his eyes. "Richard! Open your eyes!" LaPorta practically yells. "I once had a patient like this, who wouldn't wake up, and it turned out I called him by the wrong name. Then I called him by the right name and he woke right up," LaPorta says. He doesn't need to do that now, however, as Richard Arnold wakes up and the anesthesiologist can pull his tube.

Ten minutes later, with Richard Arnold once again asleep, but this time in the Recovery Room, Rob LaPorta heads down the hall toward the Anesthesia Department office and sleep.

"Dr. LaPorta?"

"Yes?" He turns back toward the nurses' station at the entrance to the Main O.R.

"We just got a call from the E.R. They've got a fourteen-year-old with suspected appendicitis. He'll be up in twenty minutes."

Tonight only patients get to sleep.

51

4:40 A.M. It takes an hour, not twenty minutes as promised, but the fourteen-year-old appendicitis patient is finally wheeled into the Main O.R. He is accompanied by his very tired, very distraught mother, who tells Rob LaPorta that her son had a cold a week ago and has been feeling sick since last night. "He complained about stomach pains and he's had a fever and been vomiting and had diarrhea," she says. "I called the doctor a couple of times, and around midnight they called back and said to bring Richie to the Emergency Room." The woman strokes her son's long blond hair as LaPorta starts an IV in the boy's right arm and hangs a bag of saline solution on the IV stand attached to the gurney.

"Richie, when did you last eat or drink?" he asks the boy.

"Not since around noon yesterday," the mother answers for her son.

"Nothing since then?"

"Well, I got him to take a little water around eight tonight."

"Is he allergic to any medications?" he asks.

"No."

LaPorta then runs down the standard list of screening questions and, when he is sure that his only problem is what is or is not in the teenager's stomach, he adds Versed, Fentanyl, and Metaclopramide to the IV line and starts down the hall pushing the gurney ahead of him. "We'll have you fixed in no time," he tells the boy.

No time is right. Pediatric surgeon Burt Parton doesn't reach O.R. 6 until 5:00 A.M. "Sorry I held you up," he says as he comes in, his hands already scrubbed. "The pediatrician called me earlier, but then he called back and said he thought we could wait. Then he called again, and here I am."

LaPorta and certified registered nurse anesthetist Jim Ryan, who was been working in Labor and Delivery and has come down to help LaPorta, have already run all their lines, working to the strains of the Temptations' "My Girl." The built-in radios in each of the Main O.R.'s sixteen rooms are usually off or kept very low. But at night, when the rooms are occupied by only the cleaning staffs, a cacophony of clashing sounds and rhythms echoes off the tile walls.

"It's just oxygen, Richie. It's not going to put you to sleep," Ryan tells the boy as he places a clear plastic anesthesia mask over the boy's mouth and nose.

"Richie, take deep breaths," LaPorta says. He and Ryan want to do a rapid induction because there may be food in the boy's stomach, so the sooner they can get the endotracheal tube in, and get him out, the better. "Okay, Richie. I'm going to give you something to go to sleep," LaPorta tells him. "Think about something you like. Do you like to go to the beach? Okay, you're going to the beach. The sand is hot and the water is nice and cool." He adds penathol to the IV to put the teenager to sleep, and succinylcholine to paralyze him. As soon as the boy loses consciousness, LaPorta pinches off his esophagus to prevent vomiting, while Ryan intubates the patient, getting the tube past the vocal cords and into position on the first try.

"Thanks, Jim," LaPorta tells Ryan, who heads back to

Labor and Delivery. "Okay, Burt, he's all yours," LaPorta adds.

At 5:10 A.M. Burt Parton begins the operation. "I want to make a nice scar," he says. He cuts inward across the abdomen at about a forty-five-degree angle, beginning near the top of the right hip. Four minutes after he begins, surgical resident Arnie Newman, who so wanted to sleep, comes into the room, holding out his dripping hands for gloves and gown. Circulating nurse Kevin McCarthy puts down his copy of the suspense novel *Red Star Rising* and helps the resident.

As Newman takes his position at the table, LaPorta whispers to McCarthy, "Shit. Now this'll take twice as long as it should, if he's gonna start teaching at five in the morning."

But things still move relatively quickly. By 5:23 Parton is telling the resident, "It's an early appy," as he pulls the appendix, which looks like a thick, pinkish garden slug, through the abdominal incision. As Burt Parton holds the inflamed appendix with stainless steel forceps, Arnie Newman ties the vestigial organ off, using a purse-string suture. By 5:35 the appendix is out and in a specimen jar on the instrument stand at the foot of the table. The teenager's pulse is 108, his blood oxygen saturation is 99 percent— it doesn't get any better than that—and the monitor shows his blood pressure to be 115 over 51. "You've got to examine twelve inches of the ileum," the pediatric surgeon tells the resident. "Feel those swollen lymph nodes?"

In another twenty-five minutes the operation is over. It would have gone faster had Parton not chosen to have the resident close. And now Rob LaPorta is trying to wake the patient. "Richie! Richie! Come on, Richie," he calls, patting the boy's face. "Come on, Richie, come home from the beach now, it's gotten cloudy at the beach. In fact, it's cold as hell. You're freezing your ass off, Richie! Come on, Richie, you don't want to be at the beach!" At 6:10 A.M., Richie comes back, gagging.

At 6:25 A.M., Rob LaPorta leaves the boy's bedside in the Recovery Room and heads, once again, for the Anesthesia office. He is too tired to see the note tacked to the cork strip on the hallway wall:

Dear staff,
   Busy night, but things under control. Instruments not packed for Rooms 10 and 6.
   Debbie.

In five minutes, another day without end will begin in the closed world of the Main O.R.

ACKNOWLEDGMENTS

That this book was written is a testimony to the willingness of three people to take an enormous risk:

Carol Hauptman, North Shore University Hospital's director of community affairs; Dr. Anthony J. Tortolani, chairman of the hospital's Department of Surgery; and Dr. Peter Walker, chairman of the Department of Anesthesia.

In my twelve-year professional relationship with her, Carol Hauptman has never tried to convince me to write about a nonevent at her institution, and, while she has certainly never invited me to write a negative story about North Shore, she has never lied to me about those negative stories I have found over the years—which makes her and the members of her staff virtually unique among the public relations representatives with whom I have dealt.

Tony Tortolani and Peter Walker were supportive of this project from the first time I spoke with them about it. Not only did they agree to my spending as much time as I wanted in the Main O.R., and not only did they not try to hide anything from me, but both men went out of their way to suggest that I poke about in departmental nooks and crannies that I might not have otherwise thought to study. For that I thank them.

Enormous thanks are also due to the dozens of men and women in the Main O.R. who went out of their way not only to not make me feel like an intruder, but to make me feel welcome in their world. They had no idea what I was ultimately going to write, yet they were willing, despite the often antagonistic view the health care professions have of the media, to take me at my word when I said I simply wanted to chronicle a day in their lives.

Thanks also to Dan Rosette, of the North Shore Community Relations staff, who responded with speed, accuracy, and good humor to innumerable requests for information about the institution.

And to Alexia Dorszynski, who established this project at Dutton, and Deborah Brody, who saw it through labor and delivery, thank you both for your endless patience, good humor, and excellent editorial direction and suggestions.

Kenneth Paul, friend, *Newsday* alumnus, and former managing editor of the *New York Observer*—and the best line-editor with whom I have worked in twenty-two years in journalism—made innumerable suggestions that only improved this book.

I appreciate all the support and forbearance I received from senior editor Elizabeth Bass and assistant managing editor Les Payne, my editors at *Newsday*.

And thanks, as usual, to Jay Acton, my agent for the past ten projects and sixteen years.

Finally, thanks to my wife, Sara Colen, always my first reader and editor. And always, the most honest.